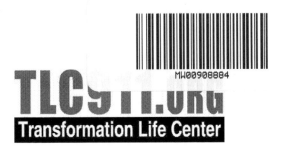
TRANSFORMED

Inspiring Stories of Freedom

"And do not be conformed to this world, but be **transformed** by the renewing of your mind, that you may prove what is that good and acceptable and perfect will of God."

Romans 12:2 NKJV

Compiled and Edited by Anita Estes

Transformed---Inspiring Stories of Freedom
Copyright © 2010
Anita Estes
ISBN 978-0-9826510-0-1

Published in cooperation with **Transformation Life Center, PO Box 249, 395 Floyd Ackert Rd., West Park, NY 12493**
Phone: 845-384-6511

All profits from the sale of this book will be donated to Transformation Life Center, which receives no government funding.

Cover design by Anita and Joanna Estes
Stories written as told to Anita Estes and Adam Popelka

Published by: Transformation House
Printed in the United States of America

Dedication

To all those affected by life-controlling issues.

To all those who have experienced God's transforming power.

Acknowledgements

First, I would like to thank Joel Sheets, the Director of TLC, for his cooperation and vision in helping to create this book. Next, I would like to thank Tom Mahairas, the founder of TLC, for his faith and determination to make Transformation Life Center a reality. Most of all, I would like to thank all the men who participated and particularly those who allowed me to interview them. It takes real courage to be honest about yourself and bare your soul. I would also like to thank Adam Popelka for securing several of the testimonies. Many thanks to Sharon Fagan for coming on board with her editing skills, along with an eagle eye secretary who wishes to remain anonymous. I thank my family for their patience with me and for allowing me to spend many hours on the laptop. I thank my daughter, Joanna, for her help with the cover design. I also thank all the administrators, teachers, pastors, counselors, and families who support the wonderful work of Transformation Life Center. Last, I would like to thank my son, Aaron, who introduced me to all these people and allowed himself to be... transformed.

~~~Table of Contents~~~

Transformation Life Center

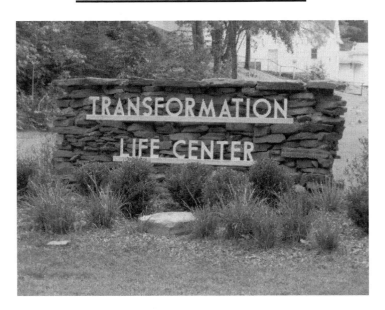

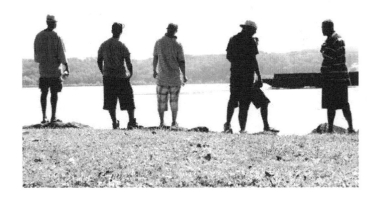

The Men

~~~From the Founder~~~

A transformed life is the greatest need of the world today. With all the brokenness and pain in people's lives, a transformed life provides hope and healing and the evidence that total change is possible. After three years of using drugs, my life was devastated. They had to give me shock treatment therapy and tie me in a strait jacket. Satan was not just a theoretical concept but had total control of my life. Demons not only controlled me, but they were using me to hurt other people. I was not only using but also selling marijuana, opium, hashish, cocaine, heroin, LSD, and pills of every kind. My life was totally self-centered.

The saddest thing about the drugs was that it was destroying every relationship in my life. I became cynical of my parents, my brother, my sister, my girlfriend, my teachers, and friends. I didn't trust anyone. It was at this time that I heard John 3:16, "For God so loved the world, that He gave His only begotten Son that whoever believes in Him should not perish but have everlasting life." That moment I put my trust in Jesus Christ and God to forgive me and to save me from all my sin. I began to read the Bible and saturate my thoughts with the Word of God. This was the key that began to transform my life. The Holy Spirit of God used the Holy Word of God to transform me into the image of the Holy Son of God. My philosophy of life was being transformed as God explains in Romans:

> I urge you therefore, brethren, by the mercies of God, to present your bodies a living and holy sacrifice, acceptable to God, which is your spiritual service of worship. And do not be conformed to this world, but be transformed by the renewing of your mind, that you may prove what the will of God is, that which is good and acceptable and perfect (Romans 12:2).

We are beggars who found bread. We want to tell other beggars where to find it. That's why we share these stories of transformation. That's why I began Transformation Life Center twenty-five years ago. We found the bread of life—Jesus Christ and want to share it with others who are hungry. We sat at the feet of Jesus and like the demoniac in Luke 8 we were transformed. Spiritually, physically, mentally, domestically, and socially we were transformed. Now we are telling others what great things Jesus did for us.

Tom Mahairas

~~~Notes from the Editor~~~

Transformation Life Center, situated in the heart of the Hudson Valley, is a beacon of hope for those suffering from life-controlling issues. It's a place of healing, restoration, and also learning. Though it is a place of refuge, it's not an escape. Rather, it's a port in the storm where men confront the issues that led to their destructive lifestyles and learn to change. For TLC is in the business of transforming men's lives through God's love, His Word, and the principles of the Bible.

TLC is also the place where guys get real about themselves and their problems, as you will read. Each one of these stories is authentic. Nothing is dramatized, Hollwoodized, or exaggerated. I know this for a fact because I interviewed the men and wrote their stories. In writing and editing, I tried to retain the flavor of their narrative in their own words. When available, I incorporated their written testimonies. These stories demonstrate in living color the power of God to redeem and transform lives once marred by the pain of addiction.

The Power to Change

If you have a family member or know someone caught in the grip of addiction, I understand what you're going through as my son's story lies within these pages. Since I know the pain and anguish of this terrible affliction, I want to offer you a lifeline—the secret behind every one of these stories. While there are many things you can do that are helpful—such as family interventions, finding a good rehabilitation facility, counseling and medication, the best course of action is prayer.

Effectual, fervent prayer is powerful. I believe it is the only thing that can really change a person's heart. For two years I pleaded with my son to go for counseling and get into a treatment center, but to no avail. While I had been praying for him for years, I started to see some real changes once I began to stand on the Word of God and thank Him for doing what it said. Let me explain.

I found a number of Bible verses that applied to my son's situation, and I prayed them on a daily basis, reminding God that these were His promises and thanking Him for accomplishing them. While I can't tell you everything I learned in just a few words, I can give you some scriptures that helped our situation. Here are just a few taken from the New American Standard Bible:

- "They should repent and, turn to God, performing deeds appropriate to repentance." **Acts 26:20**

- "And do not be conformed to this world, but be transformed by the renewing of your mind, and prove what the will of God is, that which is good and acceptable and perfect." **Romans 12:2**

- "The LORD will accomplish what concerns me (him)." **Psalm 138:8**

- "No weapon that is formed against you will prosper." **Isaiah 54:17**

- "That you may be filled with the knowledge of His will in all spiritual wisdom and understanding." **Colossians 1:9**

- "'I know the plans I have for you,' declares the Lord, 'plans for welfare and not for calamity, to give you a future and a hope.'" **Jeremiah 29:11**

- "Create in me a clean heart, O God, And renew a steadfast spirit within me." **Psalm 51:10**

- "But the desire of the righteous will be granted."
Psalm 10:24

I would pray these and other verses every day, sometimes a few times a day, and substitute my son's name in the appropriate place. After a few months of doing this, I was able to let go of my son and put him in God's hands—the best place for him anyway. I gained peace and a further trust in the Lord. After six months my son's circumstances came to a head, and he was willing to go into Transformation Life Center. He started out in the outpatient program but soon entered into the inpatient, and then he stayed an additional six months in the Residence Assistant program.

The Lord used TLC as a means to bring my son back to Him. I have often expressed my gratitude for such a wonderful program. This book is an outgrowth of my appreciation. As I saw my son's life transform in front of my eyes, I also saw other men being changed and delivered, and an idea began to grow. I thought that other people in the communities where these men live needed to read these inspiring stories. My vision for this book has expanded to include anyone who has a son or daughter or even knows someone with an addiction.

Though TLC is a unique place, the principles they use are found within the pages of the Bible, and everyone who knows God is capable of prayer.

All of the boys and men I interviewed said they had someone praying for them. So take heart and get down on your knees—anyway you can.

If you want to read more about my son's transformation and how prayer changed him, look for my upcoming book: ***Letters to God On a Prodigal Son— How Prayer and Praise Helped Overcome My Son's Drug Addiction.***

You can also visit me on my web-site at: www.anitaestes.com or write to me at: anitawriter7 @yahoo.com

From Gang Leader to God Seeker

Kayson's Story

Everyone calls me Kay—though my last name means little, I never did things in a small way. I thought I was a big shot, until God got a hold of me. Here's my story.

I grew up in Paterson, NJ in the 70's. Gangs ran rampant in my neighborhood, and I revered them and what they represented. Though I went to church with my grandmother as a child, at the age of fourteen, I decided I wanted everything the world had to offer—money, power, and prestige. I joined a gang, started doing drugs, and then dealing them. I was brainwashed by the values of the world. By the age of seventeen I was brought under the wings of organized crime and made a killing.

I was flying high—doing whatever I wanted and living in one penthouse after another in New York City. By the time I reached the age of twenty-one, I was a millionaire, supplying New York and New Jersey with enough drugs to keep me rolling in dough. I was married and had two sons who were raised to idolize me and my hard-hitting way of life.

At twenty-five, it all came crashing down on me. I was busted and sentenced to a maximum-security prison for a very long time. I watched my kids grow up from behind bars, and they saw what my lifestyle brought me to: a dead end. I wanted them to learn from my mistakes. I had gone to college but dropped out because I didn't see any reason to continue. I was making millions back then supplying drugs, but I also had skills as a carpenter and auto mechanic, my sideline career.

While in prison, I was known as a tough guy, a leader of a prominent gang who didn't put up with anyone's crap. People respected and feared me. I'd watch people die every day—fights, stabbings, being burned, you name it, I saw it. Prison has its own rules that most people will never know about. I thought I was tough and that's why I survived, but really it was God protecting me.

At the age of thirty-nine I was released on parole and promised God I would serve Him. I went back to my family and started working, two jobs in fact. I wanted to stay clean, off drugs, and I did—for a while. But then I got overwhelmed. I started using heroin again to escape; it also gave me the energy I needed to work harder. I was running myself ragged. I needed more money to get more drugs, and I needed more drugs to keep me going. I'd promised my family I wouldn't do drugs again, but I got caught in a vicious cycle.

Thirty days before my parole was up, I started dealing drugs again. I felt conflicted. I didn't want to get caught dealing and be sent away for life, but I needed the money. I knew I had to stop, but I didn't know how. My motives were all wrong.

I remember the day before Thanksgiving, I asked my wife to drop me off while I went to the store down the road. But I wasn't going to the store; I was going to make a drug deal. I met the guy a few blocks away and made the transaction. As I was walking back I noticed this white guy step into the street. He looked suspicious as he turned towards me and then asked me what I was doing. As it turned out he was from the prosecutor's office. It had been a set-up and he found the drugs on me.

I was put in an unmarked car with tinted windows, and we drove down the road past where my wife was waiting for me outside the car. My heart sank. I'll never forget the fearful look on her face. I was being taken to prison again, and she wouldn't know until she was told by someone else. I remember feeling devastated at the thought of what this would do to my family.

Back in jail, I got the drugs out of my system and got clean. Then one day I distinctly heard God tell me, "If you leave here and do the same thing, you will die." I was a little taken aback by how clear this message came across, but I told the Lord, "If you get me though this, I'll serve you whole heartedly." From that day on, I submitted to God. I experienced a radical change in my life.

I started praying and reading the Bible every night in my dorm. At this point in time I was living with seventy other guys who respected and feared me as a leader of a powerful gang. But then God did something radically different as these men realized the change in my life. I began helping any new guys who entered the facility. I gave them food, tried to get them well, and offered reassurance. I kept order in the dorm.

Other gang members wanted to know why I took these actions. I told them about God. They asked questions, lots of questions. I began leading them in Bible studies. At first for just a few guys, then more came to join. They witnessed the love of God in me. That's when I started becoming the man God wanted me to be. Not long after, God started moving on my behalf. I was facing a possible fifteen-year term, but then the courts dropped the distribution charge and changed it to possession instead. I was going to be released soon!

I called my former boss and he wanted me back on the job as soon as I was free, but my pastor stopped by and talked to me about a drug rehab called Transformation Life Center. She asked me how I'd feel about going there, and I said I'd agree to go if it's what God wants for me. She gave me the number of the intake counselor, but I never made the call. I didn't want to go through the trouble of paying for a calling card, so I disregarded the idea. Something strange followed.

Thereafter, each week the police would come down to bring me to the warden, but I had never submitted a request. I thought they were setting me up, so I made the decision not to go. After the third week of this they told me I didn't have a choice; I had to go because someone was trying to contact me, so I went. (This is highly unusual, as they don't often allow prisoners this privilege.) Anyway, they persuaded me to call TLC, and I spoke with the intake counselor.

He told me I needed some information and explained the program cost. I told him I didn't have any money, and I didn't have all the information he needed, but he persisted and asked if he could interview me over the phone. I said yes.

A week later I was scheduled to be released. It all happened so fast. Within an hour I saw the judge, and I was sentenced to three years probation. Then the papers were signed, and I was released. I was shocked, as this was usually an all day process. I didn't understand what was happening.

As the gate lifted up for my release, I stepped out and my pastor pulled up. She told me someone from TLC was here and would accept me, RIGHT NOW. I thought about the promise I made to God and said, "I'll do it." I went straight there, and I've been there for almost a year. God has blessed me so much for coming here and staying.

It's amazing what God has done in the past year. He's restored me to my wife and family. She works in the ministry at Walter Hoving Home, and we do partner ministry together. Now that I'm in the Resident Assistant Program, I can visit her most weekends. Although both my sons are still in gangs, God has mended our relationship. My youngest was the most bitter towards me because I was in jail his entire life. He has started coming to church and is learning about God. He's open to the Word of God.

God has opened doors for me both in New York and New Jersey. After I graduated first phase, I was offered a scholarship to Somerset College for Christian counseling. I've also been offered a home for my family and the chance to be part of a ministry. I was about to take advantage of one of these opportunities, but God told me to be still. So I listened and went into the second phase, one of leadership.

Here at TLC I work with a lot of guys who have just come in. I understand the drug dealer mentality, the streetwise mentality, so I just give them a big hug and take them under my wing. They need a lot of love and time to sort things out. I try to show them the love of God and lead by example. I think the guys look up to me and respect me because they know what I came from and they realize how God has changed me.

In two weeks I will graduate from the Resident Assistant phase. I'm waiting to hear what God has planned for me to do. I know people's lives have been changed by my testimony, and I'm tempted to return to my hometown, but God has been preparing me here. It was hard when I graduated from the first phase to say no to the offers, but I know I need to wait on God. In the past I was prideful. I need to let God work humility in my life. He has shown me it's not about me; it's all about him. He needs to keep me in my place. If I take a position before God wants me to, pride might pride seep in. I am aware that if that happens, I'd be done-in. So I'm careful to listen and obey. I want to do things God's way, not mine.

This is a total reversal from how I lived my life for over thirty years. I understand that's what transformation is all about. It's the power of God to change lives—from gang leader to God seeker.

Made in His Image

Vinnie's Story

As I grew up in Long Island as young boy, I had everything I wanted. When I was a little older, I realized our family was a little bit different than everyone else in the neighborhood. Our yard was bigger, our house nicer, and I had all the toys I ever wanted. There was always money around; we lacked for nothing.

As I grew a little older I heard the kids in the neighborhood saying, "Vinnie's dad's in the mob." I remember seeing the newspaper clippings of my dad with Mike Franzese who was a "made man" in the Mafia. They were very good friends, and we called him Uncle Mike.

From that point on, I started worshipping my father. I wanted to grow up and be a mobster. It was my dream to be like my dad. I started studying his habits and mannerisms. I idolized him; he was savvy, and I wanted to be like him.

When I was ten years old, my mother and father began going their separate ways. My dad was on the FBI's most wanted list and the police were always harassing him, though they couldn't trap him. The FBI used scare tactics when trying to influence him, which my mother hated. She couldn't take the threats to the family anymore, so she left with my brother and me for Jacksonville, Florida. I loved and missed my dad and became very resentful towards my mother.

My dad came to Florida, and they reconciled for a while. We moved back to Long Island for a few years, and then they separated. I was feeling bad, so I returned to Florida to be with my mom. I started experimenting with drugs to the point that I was asked to leave the high school there in Jupiter, Florida. I moved back to New York.

The same thing happened back in New York. I was smoking a lot of pot and asked to go to the alternative high school in the evening, so I did. Then I got into heavy stuff, like mushrooms, and acid—LSD. I was living with my dad and doing drugs all the time, and then I started selling them. After six months, I quit school and went to work for my dad in his construction business in Long Island. At seventeen I started experimenting with cocaine with my neighbors from my childhood.

I really wanted to try crack, but my friends didn't want me to. They tried to keep me away from it and wouldn't let any of the dealers sell it to me. Finally I got a hold of some, and it got a hold of me. I was hooked. I didn't look like I was an addict. I was good at fooling people. From the age of seventeen to thirty-one, I robbed my family and friends and lost all self-respect. At this point no one wanted to be around me, and I lost everything.

At thirty-one I wanted to join the Army. I thought this was the answer to my problems. With my record, I had to get waivers, but I managed to get them and I enlisted for three years. While in basic training, I began selling pills—barbiturates, morphine, even chewing tobacco. It seemed so easy. I remember making $4,000 in one month. I got away with a lot. At the time, I didn't realize how manipulative I was and it was becoming part of my personality. When I finished basic training, I was very proud of myself.

After basic I came home, and I couldn't wait to strut around town with my uniform. I wanted to go back to the old hood and show them how well things were going for me. Within fifteen minutes, I managed to relapse. I stayed out for three days straight, smoking crack in uniform. I didn't tell my recruiter what had happened; I gave them a story, and my father covered for me. I had to stay back an extra week so I could pass the drug test.

I was stationed at Fort Stewart, Georgia on the second of July 2006. It was one big party town, with nightclubs and bars lining the streets. The first night I got drunk, then I found someone to buy crack from. I had the money and there was no stopping me. I partied on crack for six nights.

At that point I was in the Army intake process and I hadn't been assigned a unit yet. I was very good at smoking crack at night and getting though the reception process during the day. A month later, I found myself repeating the same actions; I took my friend's Jeep, went into town, bought crack, and partied for seven nights. This lifestyle went on for seven months. Finally, I burned out and was chaptered out of the Army.

I came back home and lived with my dad. I bought a motorcycle, thinking that this was the cool thing to do and that this was the answer, but I wound up renting out my motorcycle for crack. I continued to do drugs. Finally, my dad asked me to move out. I rented a disgusting little apartment in a boarding house in Long Island. I barely existed.

One day my dad called and explained that my Uncle Mike (as we called him) was going to call me, and I was to pick up the phone when he called. He made the call and I was high, but I answered the phone. He told me that Friday he was going to set up an interview for me with Transformation Life Center. The following Monday, February 2, 2008, I was admitted to TLC. It was the best thing that has ever happened to me.

In the past, I had been introduced to Jesus at a Teen Challenge in the Bronx, but I had since fallen away. I accepted the Lord and felt the Spirit of God back then, but I gave into the flesh and Satan. Here at TLC, I have recommitted my life to Christ. God is reconstructing my life and nothing is the same.

At present, I am reconciled with my entire family. I feel that the Holy Spirit is working so much within me, opening my eyes. He is changing everything about me; the way I talk, the words that come out of my mouth, how I think, and how I act. He is opening so many doors for me, for example, college. I would like to go to a Christian college and take steps to help others. I want to become a pastor and have a ministry. My Uncle Mike, who was once a capo in the Colombo family, is now a born again Christian. He is interested in initiating opportunities for beginning ministries in other countries. I am really excited to research this opportunity.

I feel so set free now that I'm truly a Christian. My life will never be the same, now that I know the truth. I can't see myself ever going back to my old habits and addictions. Jesus has got a hold of me. I know he has good things in store for me. He performed a miracle in my uncle's life and He's now working on mine.

I aspire to be an ordained pastor, to have my own church, and to help others. My mother recently reminded me of something I said to her years ago, in the middle of my addiction, she remembered me explaining that I wanted to make a difference in the lives of other people. Even then I remember feeling God's call on my life. My dad and I don't see eye to eye on this because he doesn't know the inner transformation I've experienced. One day, I pray he will.

My dad sees only the outer changes and thinks it would be good for me to come back home and work for him. I understand this because I used to see only the outer person. Now I believe the inner person is far more important. I was always acting on my will in the past; now I want to act on performing God's will. My brother is supportive although his belief is uncertain. One day I hope he will come to the Lord.

I believe Transformation Life Center was part of God's plan for my life. This is confirmation of what the Spirit wants me to do as I continue to learn to be in tune with the Lord. I came to know the Lord in Teen Challenge but wasn't willing to overcome my fleshly desires and what I wanted (Galatians 5:16). I am now ready. I am totally in love with God and TLC has brought me to this point. I took the Word of the Lord as it's meant to be taken—to the heart. I am so thankful that my uncle recommended TLC to me. Instead of being a "made man," I'm a changed man.

A Prodigal Son

Robert's Story

There is no way to escape the will and purposes of God for your life. I was raised in a Christian home, and I believed God had a calling for my life. But I desired another way. I believed I knew better than God what was best for me, and I ran from the Lord for many years—leaning on my own understanding and trusting my own wisdom. Like Jonah, I chose a course in life contrary to God's plan, and like Jonah I ended up broken and nearly destroyed, not by a great fish, but by my addiction to crack cocaine.

The Lord blessed me, but I didn't give Him credit. I'd gone to school and obtained my Masters in Business Administration, and I had a successful career in the financial department of a large corporation. But I stopped going to church and pursued what I wanted. I had one foot in the kingdom and the other in the world. I married someone who my parents didn't approve of, and who didn't have the same Christian beliefs or morals as me. Even her friend had warned me not to get involved with her, but I married her anyway. Although she was a bank manager, she was very good at duping people. I thought I could handle what was up ahead, but I didn't realize what events would lie ahead. Even though we had two children and a nice home, she couldn't really settle down. I was just as bad. I did not honor God or give thanks for all He had given me.

Just when I thought I had achieved all my goals and was set for a life of comfort, my perfect little world came crashing down around me. My wife and I began having major marital problems. She didn't want to live up to the ideal I had in mind. She told me the only reason she married me was because she hated me, and wanted to make my life difficult. She created chaos on purpose and did things to make my mother angry. They never got along, and my mother had not approved of her or the children. Because of my wife's blatant anti-Christian behavior, my mother wanted me to divorce her and get away from the children, but I wouldn't. I felt torn between two strong-willed women. I didn't know what to do.

The stress at work also became unmanageable, and then my mother was diagnosed with Leukemia. My life was coming apart at the seams, and I was powerless to do anything about it. I should have called on God, but instead I sought escape through drugs. I'd only wanted to smoke some pot; I'd never done hard drugs before. Still when I sought out a friend who suggested crack, I didn't refuse. I thought I could handle it but found that I couldn't. I became a slave and crack was my master. This went on for years.

To the day my mother passed away, she never understood why I got involved with drugs. She never had any problems with me before, and she didn't know how to handle this. I was her only child, and she expected a lot of me. She was a strong Christian, and I felt I disappointed her. She had wanted me to go to Bible College, but I had refused and wanted to be successful on my own terms. I felt guilty about everything that happened. I had this big house by myself. My wife was a party girl and didn't really want to be a wife. I wasn't into the party scene, but because of everything that happened I chose to smoke a lot of crack, usually by myself. Eventually we both lost our jobs, and our lives spiraled downward fast.

Since I began using crack, I have lost my wife and family. I've lost my home and my career. I've been in and out of jail for various crimes and have been to several rehabilitation facilities. I never really wanted to submit to God. I wanted to live on my own terms, with my own rules. I got caught in the lies of the world. The wonderful self-centered, self-gratifying life I desired and attempted to build has come to nothing because it was built on the shifting sands of sin and selfishness.

Fortunately, God loved me while I was yet a sinner and blessed me by leading me to Transformation Life Center. He has given me another chance at life through a relationship with Him. Today I am finally letting go of my selfish ambitions for my glory and learning to seek God's glory and will. I'm learning how to submit to God. Through yielding myself to God and His ways, I have found a peace I have never known.

TLC is unique. I've been to five or six other rehabs and none are like this. Here at TLC you have a chance to come to yourself and seek God. I believe every person has to be broken to some point, to get to the place where they have no other place to turn but to God. There is no magic here, no secret formulas, just a program that gives you the opportunity to seek God. TLC helps you to come to yourself and experience the mercy of God. He is patient with us and lets us go our own way, until we come to the end of our self as I did.

Like Jonah, I am finally following the direction of God. He has delivered me from addiction, sin, and self-seeking behavior. Through Him I am learning to build my life anew on the solid rock of His son, my Lord and savior Jesus Christ. I am beginning to understand the true meaning of success. Thank you Lord Jesus and thank you TLC.

From the Bottle to the Cross

Charlie's Story

My road to addiction began a long time ago when I was in elementary school. My family moved from a rural Mid-Western town where I was surrounded by my relatives and a secure way of life. I felt lonely and confused. My parents' finances were unstable and life became uncertain. We continued to move, and it rocked my world. I turned to the bottle to numb the pain. By sixth grade I purposed to drink two to three times a week. By eighth grade I was drunk or high every day.

I continued on this path, then I quit high school and got my GED. I joined the Army and drank heavily and consistently all day long. I experimented with hard liquor and drugs, and became more addicted. When I came home, I married my high school sweetheart. She didn't know about my drinking at the time, neither did my family. I had grown up in the church, attended Sunday school, Wednesday night Bible study, and evangelistic meetings. I was able to hide it for a long time. I tried to curb my drinking, but I wound up an alcoholic. My wife divorced me.

Somehow, in spite of all of this, I was able to find my niche in advertising. I worked for Christian television and advertising agencies. Drinking was socially acceptable in these circles, and I fit right in. After a while, I could only maintain a job for a year at a time, and then I'd go back to heavy drinking. I'd wind up in jail for public drunkenness, lewd conduct, DUI's, and DWI's. This became a vicious cycle.

I was in and out of many drug and alcohol rehabs for years. None worked. Then one day my brother called me and told me about this guy, Tom Mahairas. He was speaking in Indiana, where we had lived, and was working with inner city kids. Years ago, I had helped start an inner city outreach at my church, and I longed to do something purposeful with my life again. I thought maybe I could get sober again to work with inner city kids.

At the time though, I was physically addicted to alcohol. My body would seizure if I tried to detox, but I wanted to go to this place he spoke about. I decided to take a long some help on the plane to get me from where I was living in California to TLC in New York. I hid six pints of vodka in my shirt and pants. By the time I stopped off in Chicago I drank two pints and several on-board cocktails. I had to use the men's room, and carefully placed my four remaining bottles on the floor. When I got back in the plane, I felt my jacket, and panicked. I'd forgotten the Vodka! I feared going into shock.

When I arrived in New York, two men picked me up at the airport. I was afraid I was going to have a seizure, and I shared that fear. They told me to wait and see what happened. I waited, and by the next evening, Sunday, nothing had gone wrong. I thought that was amazing! I had gone through it without a serious detox, and I didn't have to go to a hospital.

Everything was going well at this TLC. I was sober for three months, and I thought I was cured. I got ready to leave when my dorm leader stopped me and said, "When is the last time you completed something?" I thought about it. "Never!" I answered. So I stayed, and I've been here ever since.

I've done everything here at TLC, from working in the kitchen, maintenance, housekeeping, then to staff. I give God the glory for the opportunities he's opened up to me. Because of His grace, a broken down alcoholic has been restored, and I'm able to sit with respected people in the community, pastors, evangelists, teachers, and businessmen, all for the purpose of helping promote the program at TLC. Now that's God's grace.

And that's what really makes TLC unique—His grace.

Overcoming Death

Rich's Story

My drug and alcohol abuse began as a teenager—the typical hanging out, being bored, and partying with friends. It carried on into my twenties, but it wasn't just recreational anymore. I needed drugs and alcohol to get me through the day. If I had a good day, I needed to party. If I had a bad day, I needed it even more. There was always a reason to pick it up.

For twenty-five years I lived a negative, war-torn life and made it through many horrible situations. I lost my first born son to brain cancer, and then I managed to lose any money I had; I spent plenty of time in jail. Through these years my addiction got the best of me, along with my wife and kids, as well as my mother and father. I barely had a relationship with my father and sister. They tolerated me because they loved me. My mother turned her back on me to ease the pain associated with loving me and watching me destroy myself. The relationship between my wife and I deteriorated through the years, and then my oldest son was diagnosed with brain cancer. Through his battle I drank day and night to ease the pain and dull the fear of reality, but my son had faith in Jesus.

A number of months before he died, he accepted Jesus Christ into his life. He loved God with all his heart. While talking to his grandmother he explained that he spoke with Jesus about being afraid to die, and he was peaceful because Jesus would save him no matter what happened. I tried to have faith along with my son, but it wasn't real. I found myself making deals with God saying, "If you save my son, I will stop drinking." Our son died a year later.

I am not certain that anyone could possibly prepare you to watch your son take his last breath and feel his heart stop in your hand. A father is not supposed to say goodbye to his child. That night he died was the beginning of the end. I could not understand why God would take a little boy's life, especially one that loved Him so much. I cursed God with each and every drink. I wanted to die and be with my son, and didn't care that I had children still alive who needed me. I was so distraught that I caused everyone around me pain, in order that they might feel the pain as I did.

Throughout the next three years we lost everything, directly caused by my drinking and drug use. I couldn't manage to get out of bed in the morning without a drink. At this point in time, my wife took our children and left. She told me that I needed to get help before she would even consider a chance at reconciling our family. I had to heal myself from the inside, because I didn't feel that there was even a soul left in my body. I was isolated and felt completely alone, and I over-dosed from abusing drugs and alcohol.

My sister knew the wife of the director at Transformation Life Center; she advised that I get help immediately. My wife then confronted me with the ultimatum—either I go to Transformation Life Center or I would have no family. That is when I agreed to speak with the director, Joel, from TLC. He called me and convinced me not to wait any longer. He and his wife came to pick me up, brought me to the hospital, and continued sitting with me throughout the night. I went through a week of detox and then was brought to TLC.

At first, I felt useless at TLC because I was forty years old, and I felt out of place. I couldn't get the concept that I had to give it all to God to be healed. How would it be possible to love the same God that took my son? I hadn't realized at the time that there was a reason for all of this. My life then came full circle when I finally accepted Jesus Christ into my life on November 11th, 2007. I now understand that I will be with my son again. Accepting Jesus was the best thing that has ever happened to me.

Everything else started coming together when I started going to Bible studies and getting help from Grace Community Church. I am so grateful to God when I remember where I was then, compared to my life now. I am aware that my life is full and I am thankful that I have so much. I enjoy meeting so many new people that along with me, share a love for Jesus Christ. I can hardly believe I've continued to progress and recover. I have noticed that everyone now wants what I have; yet no one used to want what I would give them. I used to be a thug, and now I can lay down my life for others. I can pray with strangers that I meet in Wal-Mart. The more I can do to serve the Lord and others, the better I feel.

My son always wanted our family to be together. He wanted us all to live happily and in harmony. He was very big on going to church. I can only aspire to be half the man he was; my attitude now portrays what he always wanted. He was our precious angel. I am finally happy with myself. I am living the life that my son would have lived, if given the chance.

I continue to give it all up to God in everything I do. I realize that without Jesus, none of this would have been possible. I believe I understand the purpose for my son's life and death. My love for Jesus Christ has reached out to everyone around me, "One sheep to save the flock." This journey has been awesome. I keep going everyday by faith and to honor my son. Today my family and I are together, and I am certain that none of this would be possible without God. I was once broken; now I am healed!

Surrendering All

Ben's Story

When I was about fourteen, I started smoking pot and drinking. It started out as very occasional use to experiment with and be accepted by my peers. Then, it turned into a habit that hooked me. I started drinking more when I was twenty-one and using some coke. At first I said I would never buy the stuff and only let people give it to me. As with the marijuana, the coke use started slowly, but over a few years it grew into a full blown habit. It messed up my life really badly. I lived the street life when I knew I didn't have to be living like that.

When I was going to college in Florida, I left my apartment to go live in a gang house where there were shootings, and I slept on the floor with roaches crawling all over me. In the worst of my addiction, I was at the mercy of drug dealers to drive them around for my next fix. I still continued to believe Satan's lie that sin was better than God's goodness.

Coke opened the door for crack. Even during my coke use, I thought I would never use crack because it's "seriously dirty." I left the door ajar for Satan though, and crack crept in. There was a girl in my apartment complex who wanted to use crack at my place, and I was hesitant at first. I then let her. After being down on coke one day, she said I should use her crack, and I did. I got hooked on that too. As marijuana did a few years earlier, it caused me to have to leave college. I knew I needed to leave the situation in Florida so I moved back to New York and got clean for a while. Though, I didn't truly want to leave the life that embraced sin. I went to the bars and rationalized that drinking a few beers was okay, and I got involved with a girl immorally.

I continued to leave the door open for Satan while still "knowing" the Truth of Christ. But I had never committed to living my whole life under the Lordship of Jesus Christ. After breaking up with the girl, I used crack again for a while and finally after years of my mom praying for me and wanting me to go to rehab, I submitted to her and went to Transformation Life Center. It was the best decision I've ever made in my life—seriously. I finally committed to surrender my life to Jesus Christ.

Through TLC, God gave me the opportunity to actually live life again. Before TLC I was paranoid and oppressed by Satan and his demons. When the Bible mentions witchcraft in Galatians 5:19 as one of the obvious acts of the sinful nature, the Greek word used is pharmakea, from which we get our word pharmacy. I looked it up in a Bible dictionary, and it said the meaning of pharmakea was the magic arts and the use of drugs. Using drugs (even and especially marijuana), brings you into a realm of satanic influence.

Galatians 5:20 also mentions drunkenness as being sin. I needed to realize that because I have struggled with addiction, I can't rationalize as I did before. I was wrong to think that drinking a beer or two would be okay, and that it wouldn't lead me into the temptation to get drunk. Sometimes even though I didn't feel drunk, I was.

What I failed to do before TLC is focus on the goodness of the Lord and on His presence. In Hebrews 12 the writer tells us to "fix our eyes on Jesus Christ the author and perfector of our faith." I grew up in a Christian home and knew the Lord before TLC, but never fully surrendered my life to Him. The Creator who wrote my genetic code is more than worthy of my obedience.

The Lord has delivered me from addiction and so much more—from Satan's bondage and from the bondage of sin and death. Today I am free in Christ as I live in repentance and have true peace and joy. That's more than a fact. It's a miracle. God convicted me. "Why do you call me 'Lord, Lord,' and not do what I tell you?" (Luke 6:46 ESV)

I have been out of TLC for a while now, and the Lord continues to work in my life in a mighty way. I need to keep my focus on God and reject sin and temptation. God awaits us with open arms. 1 John 1:9 says, "If we confess our sins He is faithful and just to forgive us our sins and cleanse us from all unrighteousness." In Romans 6 Paul tells us that His grace, though, is not a license for us to sin.

God's goodness is truly so much better than anything else. Our minds can't always fathom that, but we can know that it is true. God instructs us to live a life that is built on the rock following Him, not on the sand living for our lusts and evil desires. He instructs us to repent in Mark 1:15. This means to humble ourselves before the Lord, and turn from sin to live for Him.

I've gotten involved with my church, Bible studies, and Campus Crusade for Christ. It's been a lot of fun, and it is necessary to be rooted in Christ with brothers and sisters in the Lord (Hebrews 10:25). I also continue to go to TLC every Thursday night and it's an awesome experience that truly helps my walk with the Lord.

It takes discipline and a focus on God to live for Him. It's the life He wants for everybody, and it's the only right way. In John 14:6 Jesus says, "I am the way the Truth and the Life, no one comes to the Father except through me." John 1:3 says of Jesus, "All things were made through

Him. Without Him nothing was made." It's only by the power of the Holy Spirit that I can live for God. I'm so thankful for the powerful, cleansing blood of Jesus Christ, and that He has brought me out of darkness into His Way—the Truth.

Early Release

Brandon's Story

I'm only eighteen years old, but I started using drugs at an early age. Both of my parents were addicts, but my father went to Transformation Life Center last year and graduated; he did really well. He wanted me to come here, but I didn't want to. He found crack in my room. He told me I had to get out or come here. I always argued with him. His motives were to help me, but I didn't want help at the time.

My life of drugs began when I was prescribed a barbiturate at age nine. By eleven I started drinking alcohol. This started the dark part of my life. I was prescribed medication for depression and anger, and I talked to a lot of psychiatrists. I had no sense of peace or joy. My parents got divorced when I was five and my dad was an alcoholic. Throughout high school I partied and graduated at seventeen.

After that I continued to party. I lived with friends for a little while, and then with my girlfriend for a couple of months. She was against drugs, and when she found out I was using more, she kicked me out, but she wanted to help me. She called my dad and tried to get me here to TLC. She told me to get help, but I wouldn't.

I lived on the streets for a while in South Jersey. My mom lives in Philly, and I moved in with her. She's a drug addict, and I would use drugs with her. She was heavy into crack and partying. I lived with her in a crack house. We bounced from house to house and leaned on other people. I'd stay at my sister's sometimes, but she didn't want me using drugs.

By that time my dad was in TLC. I saw how happy he was and that annoyed me, but I was curious. He came out a different person, always so happy. I didn't understand, and I didn't want to go to rehab. But God changed my heart a couple of days before I came here.

All my close relationships were broken. I called my dad. I needed help. I had nowhere to go. For some reason I said I'd go to rehab. He talked to me about God, and I listened. I felt better, and he managed to get me up here to TLC the next day.

At TLC I saw that in the past I would put on a mask and hide everything. I'd be lonely and show anger, but up here I could be more open about my past. I never could do that before. I always hid. Here, I received the most love I ever experienced in my whole life. I never had love like this. My dad had been addicted when I was growing up and my mom was a disaster. I was able to discover what my major problem was, which led to my addiction. My childhood was a mess. I'd flip out a lot and wanted to hurt myself. I'm getting better now. Every time I want to get mad, I think about His love; I should be dead.

No matter what I went though, God was faithful. Two major things happened while I was here. My second week here, I told myself I wouldn't leave here unless my family needed me. My sister said she needed my help. Her x-boyfriend, her baby's father, was abusing her. She wanted me to do something. I felt that she had been there for me, and I wanted to leave here, and I thought about doing something to the x-boyfriend. But then the people here came up to me and said the right things that made sense, and that made me want to stay. I was reminded that I could cast my worries on God, give Him the problem. He lifted the burden off my shoulders.

Soon after, my sister wrote to me and said things were good. She was able to get a restraining order against him. This was all very hard at first, but God worked. He wanted me to be still. He blessed both of us. My sister is not a Christian, but she's being receptive. God has also reconciled me to my mom, which is awesome.

God changed my heart. He's changed my attitudes; I hate my sin. I thought I could get clean and go right back out there. Now I understand that it's totally different. I don't have the desire to party. I hate partying. It sounds stupid; I had lived for that. All the things I lived for before seem so stupid now. The lifestyle I led just leads to death. I knew before I came to TLC that I could die from what I was doing to myself, and I didn't care. I'm not living for today anymore. I know I have a future with Christ. I have eternal life with Christ. My dad tried to tell me before, but I didn't understand, but now I do. He kept writing me, but I wasn't receptive. I've reread his letters, and now I understand.

TLC has helped me so much. It's given me discipline. I never had parents that would tell me what to do. Now I have a lot of rules, which at first I thought were stupid, but it's good for me. It's helped me to submit to authority. I use to hate authority. Now I'm forced to submit, and I'm trying to do it because I want to be more Christ like. I started digging into God's Word and truthfully, I never understood it before. He gave me eyes to see. The words jump out at me now, and I can't stay away from the Word.

I now know God has forgiven me for all of my sins. I realize that I don't have to live my life like I did in the past anymore. I am a new creation in Christ, and I don't have to go back and do the same destructive things. He's already won that battle for me. At TLC I have the most support I've ever had in all my life. I can tell my friends here my problems and work through them, instead of people telling me to suck it up. I wasn't good at relationships in the past, but here I have good relationships.

I've been thinking a lot about my mom while I have been at TLC. She was the victim of beatings by boyfriends because of the crowd she hung out with. Because she was a heroin addict, my mom didn't resist. She was too far consumed by the drugs to know what was going on. She couldn't take care of herself, but still she desired her children. My dad had received custody of us because she had been overdosing real often. I've been praying for her lately, and I received a letter from her. She has been mandated to rehab and she is thankful she has another chance at life—that encouraged me. A few weeks later she called and said she was willing to go into the Christian female rehab I told her about. I'm so thankful. God's in control.

In reply to some interview questions, here are my answers. My advice to young people—there's a better way to live than doing drugs. I've been there, and done that, and everything in that lifestyle leads to death, jail, or institutions. We cannot accomplish this with our own strength. If you're tired of trying, God gives strength to the weary.

My advice to parents—there's hope for your child because God has love for everyone. He has more love that we can understand. Be there for your children, give them love. Show them you care, listen to them. Extend your hand to help them, but forcing them will not work.

My greatest success is building a relationship with Jesus, going with Him. This is the greatest success anyone can have—going with JC. In the future I want to go to college and study to become a drug counselor for young kids and teens. Before coming to TLC, I went into a secular rehab program and came out worse. I want to help others not make the same mistakes. I want to be a positive influence for them.

A Long Journey Back Home
Gary's Story

My journey to TLC began a long time ago. It does not involve gangs, guns, physical abuse, or up to this point, homelessness. It's a simple story of me having the life crushed out of my being as the walls of addiction closed in. I was raised in a loving, nurturing, and Christian family. No drugs or alcohol abuse was ever around the house. Church, Sunday school, and youth groups were a constant presence in my youth. In fact I went to a Christian College outside of Boston. So, I was introduced to the Word of God early and lived around many Christians who were fervent about their love for Christ. Even with all of these positives in my life, I chose another path.

Fear, doubt, insecurity, self-loathing, failure, and anxiety were the only feelings that I ever allowed myself to give credence to and take root in my mind. I was scared of people and didn't believe in myself. I had a lot of anxiety and trouble sleeping at night. Any feelings of success, joy, or optimism were always short lived. There was always that sense of impending doom or negativity that enveloped me and kept me hostage. The bottle became my ball and chain.

The first time I drank I had stolen a bottle of bourbon from my parent's closet. I drank three-quarters of the bottle like it was iced tea. I ended up in the hospital. Thus began a slow and insidious descent into a self-made hell on earth. Every time I drank alcohol I did it to get the feeling of numbness and escape it provided. I had found a soul mate. Though God was never too far away, I started running for the next twenty years.

I was blessed with many earthly successes. I had a great education at a Christian college, held teaching and coaching positions, owned property, had girlfriends, and was respected in my community. None of this brought me any sense of joy or peace. Satan was setting me up and I was dancing with him. I was drinking daily. I did not want to think about how my family and friends were moving forward in their lives. At this point, I was miserable with what I had become. I was not worthy of the grace and mercy of God. I knew I had disappointed Him with the lifestyle I had chosen to live.

At some point I started losing things and my drinking had me drowning and gasping for breath. I found I could no longer take deep breaths. I was on the edge, daily. I lost my job as a teacher and a serious relationship ended. I stopped calling friends. After twenty years of being on my own, I moved from Massachusetts to Maryland to live with my family. Unfortunately, I had to bring my head full of insane thoughts and a self-worth that had me convinced that dying would be the best and easiest solution for a life filled with despair and a loss of hope.

I managed to be decent for a year; I worked at a hospital at night while I was waiting for a full time position to open. Then in 2006 I took another job, and I went right back to drinking. I lost the job. I wasn't upset. I figured now I could do what I want. I wasn't doing anything good. I had no goals, just drinking. It made me unemployable and unwanted in my family's home. My parents had kicked me out and rightfully so. I moved in with my sister. This is when the legal system took over.

I had gotten a DUI earlier and then got another one and spent forty-five days in jail. I was out on work release, but I lost my license so I took a job in town. Since I had a lot of court issues to deal with, counseling and community service, I worked third shift. I wore an ankle bracelet for six weeks that only allowed me to go to work and back home. Within three weeks, I failed a sobriety test. I knew I wasn't done with drinking. I lost my job, and my sister was about to kick me out, understandably so. I knew something had to change. One night in my sister's basement, I cried out to God, "What should I do?" I remembered hearing about

Transformation Life Center since I grew up in Woodstock, and so I contacted them.

The day I called TLC was the beginning of a true and meaningful relationship with God. It nurtured the last glimmer of hope that was remaining in me. It gave me the opportunity to become comfortable with who I am—my gifts and strengths and how to use them. It also helped prompt a big breakthrough. I needed to get off my high horse and realize I didn't know everything. I was judgmental and dismissive. I needed to learn how to treat people the right way. Essentially, I was spoiled. I wasn't use to denying myself, but God's discipline and love allowed me to reach out and ask for help. TLC was waiting with open arms.

Being here has restored me on the path in life that God had always wanted for me. Living in community forces you to learn how to listen and to both follow and lead in situations that arise daily. At home you can isolate yourself. Not so, here. TLC has improved my relationship with God tremendously and helped me relate better with others. I've had time to reflect on my mission in life. I've started thinking about my future again and being here has opened doors. After I'm finished as a Resident Assistant, I'll be going onto Missions Disaster Service.

Being at TLC has showed me that I do have a gift for teaching. I thought I'd never go back to being a teacher, but I teach here, and the guys like my classes. I've also learned a lot about God. You need to be willing to loose your preconceived perceptions about Him. Let God take hold of you and mold you. I wanted to dictate to God, but God wanted me to listen to Him.

If you suffer from an addiction and have given up hope, don't. You can be happy and love yourself again, if you find God. Let go of the stuff that's been keeping you in this lifestyle. Parents, the best thing you can do is pray. Then try to get your child into TLC so God can work on them. They may have to fall further than you want them to do, but keep on praying.

I thank God for allowing me to become broken! I thank God for the opportunity to be a servant in His Kingdom!

A New Purpose in Christ

William's Story

I was born and raised in Paterson, New Jersey. I started getting involved with drugs and alcohol at an early age. In retrospect, I believe that a lot had to do with the times I lived. In the 60's and 70's everything I was experimenting with was socially acceptable. The environment I lived in didn't help things. My parents did the best they could for me. When I was in the third grade, I was taken out of public school and placed into Catholic grammar school, but bad seeds had already been planted. I traveled down a path of addiction that lasted for over thirty years.

I am now fifty years old, and if I merely scratch the surface of my countless war stories and near death experiences, I could write a novel. Somehow in the middle of all the madness, I managed to stop the cycle. I got sober through Alcoholics Anonymous and people who never gave up on me. In 1991, I got married for the second time. We had been together since 1982, after I had divorced my first wife. Through my fist marriage, I have a son who's twenty-eight, but he wants nothing to do with me.

Even though my second wife and I are now divorced, she blessed me with three beautiful children: Madison, eleven, and a twin boy and girl Max and Rilee. Her unconditional love for me is the reason I'm still alive and at Transformation Life Center. My last episode almost killed me. I'd been drinking and drugging terribly since I'd lost my job at Fed-Ex after twelve years there. I didn't care about anything. I was tired of it all. My ex-wife found out about my condition through a conversation she overheard when I was talking to our daughter, Madison, the night before.

She and her sister picked me up where I was staying and brought me to Chilton Hospital in North Jersey. I was very sick and had nearly overdosed. I felt like I had a short circuit in my brain. I was stuttering and could not process my thoughts into words. I spent my birthday with the twins in the hospital, and God had me where He wanted me. Only He could have orchestrated the following set of circumstances and events that took place in the hospital.

I woke up one day to find a man, George Gartside, standing at the edge of my bed in the hospital. He introduced himself as my guardian angel. Through a series of God appointed events, my ex-wife had gotten in touch with this man. He was an intern pastor at a local church and an associate of Transformation Life Center, which he told me about. He also mentioned Jesus, but I didn't want anything to do with Him. I was Catholic, but I knew nothing of Christianity and of God. Still, I figured I had nothing else going for me, so I went to TLC.

On September 29, 2006 I found myself sitting on the stonewall behind the chapel dazed and confused at all that was going on around me. I had no expectations that this was going to work. I'd been in and out of rehabs before. Nothing worked. I didn't want anything to do with the people there, but they were different. In the other places I told them what they wanted to know. At TLC, there weren't formulas. They didn't push God or religion. They let you feel your way around and see where you fit in. After a couple of months, I felt different. So I told myself, what could I do to get most out of this program? I learned how to pray, to ask God to teach me how to work on myself, and to focus on what was going on inside myself and with others.

The atmosphere here was so different. Everyone here and at the Bruderhof was so nice, and they wanted nothing in return. They gave me unconditional love. Because of this, I learned how to be vulnerable. Before, I'd been walled up in myself for protection and survival. Now I was learning to love—myself and others. It was the end of my journey of selfish choices.

One evening, I wandered into a Bible study and I became part of it. They let me learn at my own pace. I continued to be involved, and in 2007, one year after I'd come here, I got baptized. It was a powerful experience, and it's been a wonderful journey ever since. I'm not the same person I was before. Everything I stood for in the world is the opposite of what I am now.

Now I'm satisfied to put others needs before myself. I like to help others who are coming through. I'm here to tell them their situation is not hopeless or unique. I can see beyond the smoke and mirrors because I've been there doing the same thing. My advice to them is that it's never too late to change. My best day drinking and drugging doesn't compare to my worst day being sober.

I still have struggles, but not like the ones before. Though I have a good relationship with my ex-wife and children, they are not available for me to see on a daily basis. All the would haves, should haves, and could haves, won't change that. She's remarried but we are still good friends, and I'm thankful I can see her and my children. They're not bitter towards me.

My suggestion to parents is to spend quality time with your children. Don't underestimate their ability to get involved in drugs, even if you are Christians. Drugs will come and find you. They will be exposed to it. Peer pressure will weigh down on them. Be involved and know what they're doing. Talk to your children about drugs and warn them. I didn't choose to have an addiction. It chose me. But now I'm free.

The only one powerful enough to stop me from continuing down the road I was on was God. I thank Him for allowing me and the people connected to me to persevere and endure all we've been through. I've now begun the journey that was always intended for me. I have a personal relationship with Jesus today. All I have to do is show up, be myself with all my shortcomings, and put one foot in front of the other. I am grateful to TLC, my family, and mostly God. I'm here to finish the race.

Unmet Expectations

Oliver's Story

"The consequences of every act are included in the act itself. Sin does not entail death. Sin is death."

My name is Oliver and I was born April 4, 1986. The surface of my story looks a bit different from many of the men at Transformation Life Center, but it is rooted in the same truth. I was raised in a Christian home and remember making a distinct decision to accept the free give of Salvation that Jesus Christ offers when I was seven. Throughout my life I was told that I had everything going for me. The collective "they" used to tell me I could do anything I put my mind to.

Music has always held deep significance in my life. I took piano lessons during my early years. As I grew older I moved to guitar and found affirmation from the attention that I received while singing and performing. I led worship throughout junior high and high school and was an active participant in my church and youth group. Even though people told me I had endless potential, I never seemed to follow through with my commitments.

As I became more fickle, this supposedly endless potential went untapped. I felt as though all of the things I was able to do kept me from choosing any one thing to pursue with all of me. I began to seek others acceptance in a more urgent way. I felt helpless and there was an angst building inside of me that told me I was not measuring up; not living up to peoples' expectations. As I allowed myself to let commitments and promises go by the wayside, I caused these angst driven fears to become reality. In the next few years my worship changed. I was singing for me to feed the need inside me. I walked away from the Master and surrendered myself to less passionate lovers.

I did not take my first sip of alcohol until I was nineteen. I was not even exposed to the partying scene until after my senior year of high school. I can remember the first time I poured myself a drink. I acted cool, collected, experienced as I poured a drink for Bree, my girlfriend at the time, and myself. The sun was just below the horizon, and I can still hear the sound of the carnival outside of the window. It was innocent and happy and had a distinct feel to it; it was something resembling home. It was twisted and dark, and poisoned beneath the surface, though it was some time before I was able to see this as the truth of the matter.

Bree played a strong role in my opportunity to wander off the path. She presented me with what I considered to be a viable excuse. I wanted to be with her. She gave me meaning. She was versed in the nuances of this dangerous lifestyle, and I too wanted to know. I wanted to possess the savvy and mystique she personified.

The sweetness on my tongue would turn sickly in my stomach, but all of the things that attracted me to this lifestyle were still too avant-garde to discourage my fervor. I began to neglect the things that I enjoyed, and the people whom I loved. I made manifest the negative disposition I used to project on myself. The things that gave me the desire to try this road now perpetuated my need for it.

I felt I had no hope and became numb to the truth about myself. My talents went unpracticed. My studies were maltreated. I felt acutely inadequate, but instead of going up for air I went deeper. My girlfriend was the door to this realm of novel excitements and I had not even begun to quench my thirst. I lost myself in her and the life that she represented. My personality was changing. I watched myself become reclusive and melancholic, but I was indifferent. I stepped forward, yielding myself to my desires.

I proceeded to augment my selfishness and depravity so cleverly disguised as a throwing off of the restraints that bound me to responsibility and order. I would drink to escape people and problems. I would spend time with Bree, giving more and more of myself to her. I began to root my security and significance in her solely. She was my solace. I was fully incapable of facing any type of responsibility in my life. In conflict I would run; presented with decisions, I would freeze. I could no longer see anything good in me. I looked into the mirror with loathing.

At the depth of my dissolution I got into a serious accident in my father's car that I had taken to see Bree. I careened off of an embankment to an over-pass road and landed the car in a heap on its roof. This would be my second offense for driving while intoxicated and I felt debased. I sat on the hill virtually unscathed, the vodka losing effect. In the cool of the early morning, after limping away from the ravaged driving machine, I knew that this was it. I was going to have to face myself and give an account.

My probation officer was a follower of Christ. She was the catalyst that brought, or rather forced, change in my life. I knew I needed to escape. I had no idea how I was going to achieve this. I was not brave enough to take one step. I knew that I must be taken far away from the sirens' luring call, if any type of redefining was to be done in me. My aunt found Transformation Life Center online and shared it with my mom. Quickly, my probation officer made the preparations. I was willing because I had to be—anything but jail. In two days time I was gone from everything and everyone I knew. What I was not aware of at the time was this—that man would never return.

Initially, I believed I was where I needed to be at TLC. I knew I would stay there for a full year, I had been ordered to do so by my probation officer. The exterior of my story, however, differed so much from the other residents that a division formed in my mind. Many of the residents would ask me what I was doing at TLC, the "perfect church boy."

I was encouraged by the leadership and supported by friends and family at home. They reminded me that I was at TLC for such a time as this. The other residents' arguments and accusations quickly faded and determination replaced any doubt. I was going to do what I had to do. So, requirement turned to resignation, resignation to a willful decision, a decision to personal resolution, and resolution to graduation.

After the first six month phase, I stayed on for the second phase. Once completed, I had succeeded in putting one year between my transforming self and the man I used to be. Transformation Life Center became the grounds on which I was able to escape my nightmare and come face to face with my true self. I learned who I am.

During that year I learned that my most deeply rooted fear was that of rejection. This was the root of all my anxieties. If I was not fulfilling others expectations, I felt alienated. Upon learning these truths about myself, I started to see in me who I was before my digression. Without Bree, without alcohol, without the party, I slowly began to see confidence, enthusiasm, courage, optimism, creativity, joy. These were my qualities, I was remembering.

Today I enjoy and embrace who I am. This walk I am on is not about some super-spiritual monastic religiosity; it is about life. It is not about what you did, but what you will do. It is not about who you are, but who you can be. My future is now.

As a result of what the Master has done in my life at TLC, I know my potential. I am once again using my music to offer an oasis of worship to those around me. I am involved in Sunday services and small groups. I am in community. I am a part. I am involved with a purpose. I am caught up in a story greater than myself. I am filled and I have given myself to the Master in total abandon.

My priorities have completely changed. Before, I felt hopeless and worthless. I had no direction. Now, I seek God to show me the way. I seek Him to do as I ought to do for each day. I pray and I depend on God. People, look for His will—*do as you ought*. Do what His love letter to you tells you to do. It is a guide for fullness in life. It is a passion promoter. He makes me more who I am each day.

What is required of you in your daily life? Are you

satisfied by it? Day by day I give over more of myself, and I long to grow in the knowledge and grace of the Master, Jesus Christ. As I seek Him, my path is defined and my way is straight. There is no question. He is the way I will go.

I hope my story reaches those of you who are in the thick of the dark forest that I described in the beginning of my story. If you have any depravity in your life, whether it is a dependency to alcohol or drugs or simply the emptiness inside you that nothing will satisfy, I know where you can find the freedom you crave. You must to be ready to have all you think you are stripped away. Know this: whatever you think you have is a lie. It is your bondage, not your savior. The very things that you feel are protecting you are those which are draining your life.

The hope I found is in a relationship with Jesus Christ. He has taught me to understand my purpose. He showed me the path for my life. He will do the same for you. Do not allow your passions to be sapped by less passionate lovers. The creator of the universe died for you. The one through whom everything exists gave up all He had to save you. If you think you have nothing, know that the one who is Love can show you who you are. He is throughout, above, and beyond all of the expectations I had.

In His Hands

Ralph's Story

My name is Ralph. In August of 1983 I was born in Pequannock, New Jersey. I was the first grandchild and the only child of my parents, that reserved the right to be spoiled, or so I thought. Being that my home was broken, growing up was very unsatisfying. My mother and father were using drugs themselves so it was very difficult to find satisfaction as a young child with either of them. All I could remember about my childhood up to age five was constant fighting resulting in emotional abuse, habitual parties, and always being alone.

By the age five my mother's addiction and desire for other men ruined my parent's marriage. After the divorce my father brought me to live with his parents. I lived with my grandparents from age five to sixteen years old. Needless to say, my grandparents were very well established and spoiled me with everything and anything I wanted. During my teenage years I struggled with acceptance. I looked for affirmation from women and friends in all the wrong ways. During those years I experienced many trials; after growing up in a broken family, I never experienced the security of a functional family.

Seeking affirmation from all types of people with different backgrounds, I finally fit in with the last group and got into wrestling and smoking weed. I became very popular. I looked for affirmation from them and the attention of women. After high school, I went to Centenary College and was on their wrestling team, in which my freshman year I achieved the All-American Award. After a bad car accident, I left Centenary and went to Bergen Community College and continued wrestling. After coming home I destroyed my brand new car.

While I was in the hospital, I started selling pills for my aunt who worked in the hospital. I made a lot of money doing this, and I started taking them for myself. I fell in love with how they made me feel. I felt confident and didn't need other people's affirmation like I had in the past. My insecurities went away. After eight months, my aunt cut me off from the supply. By then I was hooked and strung out without them. I ran through all my money and started stealing from my father's bank account. After I got caught he gave me an ultimatum—either go into rehab or into the military. I chose the military.

I did well for a year. I was off drugs until one day I had to get my wisdom teeth pulled. The dentist prescribed Percocet, and before I knew it I got right back into the habit. I was taking up to a hundred a day. I got caught with them in the military and was discharged, so I went to live with my girlfriend in Florida, while she was enrolled at Nova Southeastern in a doctoral program. While I was down there I found a friend who introduced me to crack, and I continued with the painkillers.

Now I had a crack habit besides needing painkillers, which I would get from writing prescriptions on a stolen pad. My girlfriend, who was studying to be a doctor, was oblivious to it for a while. I was good at hiding things. I continued like this for a couple of months until she suspected and confronted me about the drugs. I said I would stop. At this time, she was unhappy with the school she was attending and wanted to move back up North. We decided it would be good for both of us, and we went up North to visit her parents in New Jersey and look at apartments.

While we were in New Jersey, I started going through withdrawals. Knowing my girlfriend's father was a doctor, I stole his prescription pad. I was good at imitating doctor's signatures, and I wrote out some prescriptions, but the pharmacy knew her father. It was then that I got caught at my game. I was charged with two felonies—impersonating a doctor and forgery. I went to jail and then to a twenty-eight day program. My girlfriend was there for me and packed up my things in Florida.

While down there, she found paperwork that I had gotten kicked out of the military. She hadn't known that beforehand and she was upset, but still stayed with me. She took me to the rehab and hoped I would change. While I was in the rehab, I had a yearning to know God to fill the vacuum in my heart. I had used my girlfriend to fill that void. After nine months of clean time and holding down a job with Otis Elevator as an elevator mechanic, my girlfriend and I broke up. I saved roughly $20,000 for a condo while I was clean and working. I ran though all the money I'd saved up (in three months) and squandered it on drugs.

I moved back with my dad. He felt bad for me because my girlfriend had left me, but this gave me the opportunity just to do more drugs. In the spring of 2008, my grandmother sought out an Overcomers meeting for me at Jacksonville Chapel in New Jersey. Through them she found out about Transformation Life Center and recommended I go there. I didn't care, and I didn't want to go. My father told me I needed help, but I told him I had too much to do. I said sarcastically, I wouldn't go unless someone died. Unfortunately this happened.

The circumstance that allowed me to realize how broken I was took place a month before I came to Transformation Life Center. I was with my cousin and we were both broken, looking for someone or something to save us. We were at a point in both of our lives where we were desperately in need. Being utterly distraught and very confused, we both turned to drugs. On one occasion, unguided and misled, we got together and tried heroin, trying to escape the torment of our everyday reality. That night my cousin died of an overdose. This was undisputedly the worst thing that has ever happened to me in my life.

Not wanting to deal with his death and not understanding why I was still alive, was confusing and very stressful. Not knowing where to turn, numerous manifestations of suicide attempts played out in my head. My last day at work in utter distress, I climbed to the 27th floor of a building I was working at in Manhattan with the intent of suicide. While I was up there staring down into an empty elevator shaft, all I could think about was my foreman—he and I had an excellent relationship, and I knew he would lose his job if somebody died on his shift.

I feel that God had planned that all out because that is the only thing that kept me from stepping off the ledge. That day, I came home and reached out to a man at my church who directed me to TLC. My grandmother's prayers had been answered. In June of 2008, I finally went to Transformation Life Center. Upon arrival I was not very impressed with it, but through many struggles and help from staff and other residents, I found what I had always been looking for—Jesus Christ. I felt God's presence at TLC. I had never felt such a comforting connection before in my life. I went home on pass one day, and I was looking forward to coming back. I felt like an alien in my own town and saw things through different eyes. At TLC I've gained a relationship with God, and had the opportunity to complete a one year commitment I had made. (I have never completed anything in my life.) I've had the opportunity to experience love by becoming vulnerable and transparent with other brothers, by allowing myself to be loved, and loving others.

I have never found such peace and purpose like I have since I've been at TLC. I have forgiven my mother and everyone who wronged me simply because I have accepted Christ's forgiveness and His gift of love. My life has completely changed. God has forgiven me everything I did and given me hope. I try not to look too far ahead in the future but live each day for the Lord. I'm thankful for the prayers of my grandmother who brought me to the Lord. I know it must be very difficult for parents to experience their child living a life filled with drugs, but there is hope. Prayer works. God never lets us go, and I am very grateful for that.

Drinking in God's Grace

Joe's Story

I was introduced to alcohol at four years of age, though I grew up in a strict family. At eight years old my siblings and I would clear the table, and I would fight with my brother to drink the beer left over; all the while my father was watching us. I didn't like the taste of beer, but looking back I was in an environment that constantly exposed me to alcohol.

I remember that at the time it seemed important to me to do what the other kids were doing, and the other kids were usually partying. Hanging out with the wrong crowd was great fun, and it was then that I started partying. Hanging out with my friends and partying were good times, until it became a nightmare. But I was resolved to drinking, no matter what the outcome.

I loved drinking. I loved the ritual that came with drinking: buying the booze, ordering the food, and all the rest. I was proud that I could drink anyone under the table. However, my drinking addiction led me to the introduction and love of cocaine. I had a good job, a roof over my head, bills were getting paid, and I was using the advancements on my pay to buy coke. From the age of twenty-four to twenty-nine, I abused cocaine. I believe genetics might have had something to do with my addiction to alcohol; science might prove that. However, I don't blame my compulsive behavior on anyone in my family. Being compulsive is just a part of my nature.

There was a point in time when my life started spinning out of control, and it was noticed by everyone around me. I remember thinking that it was just a phase and this behavior would soon pass. By the time I was twenty-three years old my life was full-blown out of control, although I didn't realize it. I was in denial and I had no outside help involved; however, I wasn't seeking help and none was offered. That Christmas, at age twenty-four, my brother gave me an Alcoholics Anonymous Big Book. I am certain that my family had no idea how to help me, so their effort resulted in just a Big Book thrown my way. It seemed to me that my family felt that this book was the world's end-all answer to the problem they noticed I was having. Eventually my boss approached and confronted me, discussing the fact that I had a coke problem.

I managed to quit coke by becoming a twenty-four hour a day drinker. I only used coke when people offered it, and I eventually quit. At this point, I was drinking all the time. I switched my choice of drink often, as I believed that by switching drinks I would keep my addiction from being too noticeable. My wife, Elena, who was my girlfriend at the time, picked up the scent of whiskey on me too often, so I switched to white wine and wine spritzers. Each day my drinking started when work was over. But on my days off, the drinking began as soon as the day started. My drinking hadn't resulted in me shaking, yet. However, I am sure that I was unapproachable for anyone to tell me that I had a problem. Because of this, my life was reduced to living alone in the woods. I had nothing to my name. I'd make an attempt to go to a detox just to sleep in a bed. That is when I truly started to realize that I had a problem. I thought that I could either continue not to care, or decide to get help.

The first time my wife convinced me to attend my first AA meeting, I went just to keep my marriage from ending up in divorce, not because of my drinking. I stopped drinking because I didn't want to lose what little I had around me. I like to drink; if I could drink today, I would, but I cannot drink without getting drunk. I don't drink to help my steak digest; I drink for the effect.

Many times I tried to quit on my own and attended outpatient programs, resulting in some success. Before I found the Lord, I had a total of six years clean and sober. I picked it up again and went for a year and a half run, though my whole life came apart within the last six months.

One day I walked an exhausting journey from Paramus, New Jersey to Jacksonville Chapel to try and get help. They helped get me to a detox and then to Transformation Life Center. I wasn't looking for Jesus or salvation, although my heart wanted to complete a year there. I desired to stay forever because of the situation at hand—divorced and no job. I had gone to TLC with nothing, and soon after I had enough clarity to realize that staying was much better than going back to a tree in the woods.

My wife reconciled with me while I was four months into the program. She asked if I would stay for the second phase. As much as I wanted to go home, I knew that because of our finances and our relationship, I needed to stay to finish my commitment. I would have picked up drinking again if I had only stayed for the first six months.

There were a lot of rough times when I first got home. I felt guilty and ashamed because of what I had done in my previous life. I had the Lord's forgiveness and my wife's forgiveness, but I still felt like I didn't belong. I was afraid that I wasn't the perfect Christian. My wife and I walked on eggshells (in her words), hesitant to say anything that might result in setting me off and drinking again. I wasn't capable of keeping the promise to never drink again. My wife was never able to help get me clean or help keep me clean.

I have the best chance of remaining sober by clinging to Jesus. I have my challenges and think about drinking every now and then. I think about having a Sam Adams. Then I am reminded of what could happen with something as minor as having a beer. I approach the Lord with my problems, and He answers. It is so nice not to have to worry about going to bed when the birds start singing, or where to find my morning bottle of booze. I am so blessed!

After completing TLC, I felt like I never really left. I went to TLC's Thursday night Praise and Worship service every single week for eight months after I graduated. Sometimes, it sucked after coming home from TLC because I felt like the only thing missing from Joe was a bottle of whiskey. Sometimes my behavior didn't change at all. Living life on life's terms is very difficult. Things are hard outside of TLC. Life isn't easy, but now I have the Lord to help. I try to stay in line with what the Lord says in His Word.

I raise my hand to whatever comes my way within the Lord's biding, but I have to be in line before I can do what He asks of me. I raise my hand to keep myself from falling back and drinking. I must be in check before I can let the guys from TLC come stay over my house when they go to participate in doing community awareness in New Jersey. I must be still and wait on the Lord, but that doesn't mean that I can be lazy. I cannot say that I am waiting on the Lord and do nothing. I have to do what I have to do. Now, when I get frustrated, I take a step back and look at my wife. I look at my daughter, Jess, and remember how blessed I really am. The key for me is not to worry about what other people think, but be concerned about what the Lord thinks. I fall short every day, but the Lord delivers me from sin. Through Him I can talk to God.

I must be accountable to the Lord, and for all the service related things He has me doing for other people. I am blessed in serving and helping others. What's the blessing? I didn't use alcohol or drugs for that day. Does that mean I have no other sins? No. If I was totally delivered from alcohol, I wouldn't have to stay involved in all these activities; they help keep me from sin and it keeps me clean. I attend the Overcomers in Christ meeting weekly at Jacksonville Chapel in New Jersey. I've been so blessed. I can now go back to TLC, see my bed, remember my time there, and what God has done for me—like giving me some of my greatest desires. It's so great that I get to do something I really like—playing the bass guitar with the worship team at TLC. It's amazing. God has completely turned my life around.

A Life of Second Chances
Raul's Story

I grew up in West Virginia with a father who was a drug addict. When I was young, my mother and father divorced and my mom remarried. Though I had a lot of freedom when I was younger, my new step-father imposed a lot of rules. He was very religious and I had to attend church, Wednesday night Bible study, and evangelistic meetings.

Then my step-father went to Bible College, and the family moved on campus with him. He became even more restrictive, and I grew to resent him. I was forced to go to meetings and listen to many testimonies. Though I intellectually accepted Christianity, I was attracted to sin. I lived in a sheltered environment in West Virginia, and I wanted to have fun. Though my body was in church, my heart was in the world.

In high school I didn't drink much, but when I joined the Marines I started drinking regularly. I was using it to medicate myself from what was happening around me. When I got out of the military, I went to Seminary School. Then my real father died violently. He had been a heroin dealer and was murdered. I fell apart, and started seeking hard drugs. Everything totally disintegrated. I didn't have a good relationship with him, and I hated him for being absent when I was growing up. This resentment festered.

After my father passed, I left school and got involved in psychedelic drugs and Eastern religions. I sought mystical experiences through these drugs and expanding my mind. I wound up working in a recording studio in Cincinnati and had access to any drug I wanted. Then my grandfather died and left me money. I took my inheritance and bought a house in Pensacola, Florida. I squandered the rest on drugs, so I started growing my own mushrooms and pot, as well as extracting peyote from cactus. But God still had His hand on my life. All my neighbors were Bible college students, pastors, and teachers. They invited me to Bible studies, meetings, and church; and I went.

One day I was in my house alone. My roommate, who smoked crack, had just stolen my car. I was feeling very depressed and suicidal. God put me in a corner and I couldn't move, like a chess piece trapped by his own poor moves. I felt convicted, and I cried out to Him. I called my family and asked for help. I threw out the drugs in the garbage, but unfortunately I retrieved them later, even though I meant to stop using them. I was ready to go to rehab, and I did. I went to a thirty day program in Phoenix. I stayed clean for a while.

The first year of being clean was really difficult. I was a shift manger at Papa John's and everybody there was smoking pot and doing drugs. One day, I stepped into a Baptist church and they were having a prayer meeting. I joined in and started going there. Eventually, I moved back to Cincinnati with my family and went to church with them. I worked locally at a Teen Challenge Christian Rehabilitation Center and as a full time youth minister at my church. It turned out to be too much too soon, as I was too young in my faith. Even though I was enthusiastic and had a passion for holiness, I had doctrinal issues with my church. They decided to send me to college at Word of Life Bible Camp in upstate New York.

At first I worked at the Inn and went to college. They made me a tutor for seven young Korean women, which wasn't a good idea. Though I remained pure, I was bouncing around from relationship to relationship. It was a problem. Their attention fed my ego in a negative way. I lied about my relationship with them. God told me I was running from Him and nothing good would come of me if I continued. I didn't listen.

I was questioned by the director and lied to him. The day after, I went out and got drunk, stole some things, and bought alcohol. I stayed drunk for a few days. They sent me home for a few months, and then I came back to Word of Life. Things became worse. It was obvious that I spent most of my time ripped to the gills. Understandably, I was kicked out. I then entered into a program in Albany and completed a nine month program.

Everything was going pretty well there. I was working in the clinic, but I felt I wasn't getting paid enough so I started selling drugs. Not only was I dealing them right from the facility, I was growing them in a secluded section of the building. No one knew. I had a thriving business. But I started feeling guilty, so I talked to the director about it. The both of us destroyed everything I was growing— mushrooms, pot, and cacti.

Under his advice, I went away for a week and then came back. They told me I no longer could come back and work, so I found another job. I tried to get back into ministry, but couldn't. I wasn't doing well. On top of it, my ex-girlfriend had re-lapsed, and then my good friend died. I relapsed and drank for two weeks straight. My pastor put me into Transformation Life Center.

TLC has helped me get my relationship back with the Lord. When I was working at Teen Challenge, I felt close to Him, but then it dried up. I felt it was more about religion than about God. When I got to TLC, I sought repentance like David in Psalm 51. "Have mercy on me O God, According to Your loving kindness...For I acknowledge my transgression, and my sins are always before me. Against You, You, only have I sinned, And done this evil in Your sight" (Psalm 51:1-3).

One day I remember walking into the chapel and praying this prayer. I hadn't softened my heart in a while. Finally, I cried out to the Lord, and I felt his tangible presence. It's taking me time to get back into relationship with Him. It's a process, but I'm on the right road.

I've realized that because of what Jesus has done, we can go into the presence of God. We can seek and find true spiritual experience. We can sit in the presence of God, which changes people. I thank Jesus for the opportunity to know God in this way. Now I can learn to reflect on God and do whatever He does. It has been an amazing opportunity to be at TLC. For me it's no longer a rehab, but a community of Christians serving each other— though in some ways it's almost monastic.

You can get as close to God as you want. Sometimes I might not like it, but it has definitely been beneficial. It helps you confront yourself and your problems through counseling, but most important are the relationships with the other guys. In the world we tend to isolate ourselves a lot. Living in community drags you out of yourself, which is a good thing. We need to learn how to relate to others, which is usually difficult for addicts.

Another problem is that addicts are good at manipulating others, especially their family. My advice to parents who have a child with an addiction problem is to learn to love your child properly. Don't enable them. Let them take their lumps in life; let them fall. Don't let them live in your basement and continue in this dead end lifestyle. Addicts learn how to pull on their family's heartstrings. Keep praying for them and seek godly counsel. Try to get them into a program, like Transformation Life Center.

TLC has helped me in so many ways and has provided a place where I don't have to worry about what's going on outside in the world and provide for myself. I now have ample opportunity to deal with interpersonal relationships. It has required me to be in Christian community where everyone plays a role and has fostered development of my gifts. I have been taught how to pray again. Most of all, I am brought back into a godly lifestyle because of my relationship with Jesus. I pray that I'll be able to stay within God's boundaries of grace, and not let my pride pull me under.

Redemption

Salvatore's Story

As a young boy I had a difficult time growing up. I was picked on, ridiculed, and generally not well liked. In my eyes, everyone reviled me. It may have been more my perception than reality, but I was lonely and always afraid. My life was governed by my trying to avoid people. Other children would push me around, and I'd get in trouble for it. My parents would get upset with me, "Are the teachers lying?" they asked. The problem was groups of kids would lie to the teacher, and so I was found guilty.

As an adult (who worked in a school) I now realize the flaws in the system. However, as a pre-teen I abhorred anyone in authority. I also remember spending a lot of time separated from everyone. I was the one in trouble, but I was happy to be alone and safe. The teachers always gave me books to read, and to their surprise I devoured them. They would give me higher level reading to keep me busy, and they discovered I had a great aptitude for comprehension. However, I was the villain in this story and there was no hero type who wanted to take me under his wing, but a mentor might have changed me.

At the age of eleven, I decided to wage war. It was me against them. I was smart enough to be dangerous and I became the general. I would no longer take orders from anyone. I grew a lot the summer between sixth grade and Jr. High School. I had my first girlfriend, cigarette, beer, drove my first car, and thought on was on my way. I had a best friend named Jimmy, though our parents didn't want us hanging around together. We spent the summer together; we did everything together, despite our parents. Jimmy and I later became partners in crime … literally.

At the very beginning of the seventh grade school year, I mopped up the schoolyard with the first kid who looked at me wrong. My fate was sealed. I would never be subject to anyone again. The only way anyone would get within arms distance of me was if I needed them to; I had no idea how lonely life was really going to be.

I spent Jr. High and high school chasing girls and doing drugs. I was smart enough to pass classes without ever doing much of anything . . . this included not showing up much. I had great potential, but I would waste it doing as little as possible. I had an aptitude for music, and I actually learned a bit about playing a few instruments. Unfortunately, I squandered that gift. I would only stick to things I could do immediately. I had no time to "waste" to develop anything. I didn't even finish high school in a traditional fashion. I was short some credits so I went into a program in which I could get my GED and graduate with my class. I did not attend graduation. This is one of the things in my life that has made me feel less than others. Only recently am I back in contact with some of the people I went to high school with. Even after all God has done in my life, I still find myself a little intimidated. After all, the only thing I really excelled at was underachievement.

Right after high school I married my first wife. I believed I was doing the right thing; it was a disaster. I was not even able to take care of myself, let alone a wife and daughter. My parents shouldered so much of this part of my life, and it was not until many years later that I even realized this fact. The only thing right about the whole thing was bringing my daughter, Jennifer, into the world.

Divorced after three years, I lost custody of her by the time she was eleven. In the last fifteen years, I've seen her for only a brief couple of weeks when she was fighting with her mom. I helped them patch it up and have not heard from her since. I know she has no idea how my heart aches to be part of her life, but I understand why her mother doesn't facilitate a relationship with me.

I was not a good husband in any sense of the word, so the fact that Nancy left me is no surprise. We were so young and knew . . . well just about . . . NOTHING! I often pray for her; I hope her life is rich and full. I pray for Jen a great deal. I pray they will find their way to God. I look for Jen online. I keep hoping one day we will find each other.

Anyway, moving on . . . after separating from my first wife, I became a drug dealer. I sold large quantities of cocaine and ended up using more than I sold. I have a deviated septum larger than two centimeters and smoked enough of this substance to kill an army. The fact that I'm alive and still retain my faculties is a miracle. God is so merciful.

During that time, my brother helped me pack up my little den of iniquity. We put everything I owned in a U-haul, and he helped me get ready to move in with a friend. I thought this was the end of that era, but later that night we had some visitors. This episode ended in a stalemate . . . a group of us gathered in a small apartment, some of which were holding very large firearms; the kind of situation whose aftermath usually makes the nightly news . . . did I mention that God is so merciful?

After some coaxing from my dad, I moved back home. The education I had gotten from my misadventures; while enough to slow me down, did not bring me to my senses. I was still chasing my own gratification. I got my old job back working six overnights a week. For the better part of a year, I tried to stay out of trouble. I smoked pot every day, but at that time it was as much a part of my makeup as smoking cigarettes. I never took to drinking but I smoked like a chimney.

I met my second wife working that overnight job. At the time she was in an abusive relationship, but she wasn't married. She had two daughters, one and three years old. She left him; we dated, moved in together, and eventually got married. During the reception, I found out something terrible about my good friend, Jimmy. Even though we had drifted apart, it was difficult for me when I heard he killed himself. He was all coked up, depressed, and on the phone with his mother when he took his own life with a rifle. It was a difficult way to begin a marriage, but anyway, I filed the paper work to make the two girls my legal daughters, and we began our life together.

Once again, I was not a good husband. It was not for the lack of trying, but trying is not the same as doing. There is so much I never learned. I've heard that "try as you might" you cannot do what you have not learned or been trained to do. Don't misunderstand; I had much knowledge, but no discipline. I had no idea how to understand or relate to people, or how to be corrected. I had many ideas . . . all wrong. Even though I had taken control, or so I thought, of my life, I had become a victim—always looking at the negative. That was hardest thing for me to overcome. It took me, with God's help, months and months to break through that barrier! I still catch myself at times.

Soon we had a third child, a son. My wife stayed home with the children and I worked. I started my own business at that time and did pretty well. However, I could not manage money well so our finances were a continuous struggle throughout our marriage. We managed to find our way to a Christian church. We were very involved and eventually became members. Even our children were very involved. Though I found a church, I did not find God. I can't speak for the hearts of my family, because...what did I really know about them? I was more concerned with being in charge, following the rules and worrying about whether or not everyone else was doing what they should.

I did not understand people. It has been the ruin of my life. I was very involved in the church, but that was my MO. I did not know how to have a relationship, so I would keep busy and concern myself with being "important" or so I thought. People don't remember what you have done as well as they remember how much you cared and showed love. I did manage to put together a few sober years during that time. However, it mattered not—clean and doing everything wrong . . . is still doing everything wrong.

The Bible was my biggest problem. I was the worst kind of fanatic. I stuck to the letter of the law. I beat my family half to death with it. I devoured the Word because I could, and used it like a club for my righteousness. I was a scary person. I was more concerned with what they were doing than how they were doing. I would walk into a room and see the "tasks" not the "people." I thought I cared so much. I thought I was being so diligent, but I was a tyrannical madman. I was so often right in the worst way. I could never understand why I was pushing people away. The truth is that I was always pushing. I never tried to draw anyone to me. When I tried to show that I cared, it was too little too late. Did I care? Of course I did, but as in my younger days of misinterpreting, it is the perspective of the recipient that matters. If they did not feel loved, than whether or not I showed love or not, is a moot point.

I was such a self-righteous mess, and then I went and had an affair. I never thought I could hurt someone so badly. I don't know why my wife forgave me and asked me to stay with her. I have come to a point in my life where I can understand forgiveness and am beginning to understand love. I can only assume that my wife was far beyond me in that area. Women usually are. As for the woman I had the affair with, I can't even imagine the mess I made of her life.

During this time I was injured and had to go on disability. I was home all the time and on painkillers and muscle relaxers. This was the beginning of the end. I created an atmosphere of animosity and apathy. Until this day, I don't know how my family put up with me for the better part of a decade. I also don't know how I survived eating approximately 25 painkillers and 25 muscle relaxers a day for most of that time. The mercy of God truly is new every day.

By then I realized I had a problem and wanted to stop, but when I tried my problem became very noticeable. The detox was terrible and I fell completely apart. My family and my church came together and got me up to Transformation Life Center. I went through the program and graduated Phase One in January of 2004. I should have stayed, but I wanted to go home and help my family. I felt guilty; I wanted to help them. I thought I needed to save my world. I hadn't even got my own life on track in those six months. In fact I spent those six months lying and behaving the same selfish way I always did.

I went home, got a job, found us a place, and tried to put my life back together. However, I did not learn how to do this. I ended up in a depression, out on sick leave. Every day I thought of taking my own life, but I knew just enough about God to realize how useless that would be—

outpatient at a psychiatric clinic and back on meds, this time psych meds. Well, this seemed all too familiar. My wife was so done with me at this point. The strange thing was I had really been trying to reach her, and somehow I could not bridge the gap. I had wasted so much time trying and trying, but I was unwilling to take the time to learn or develop some skills or tools that might help me achieve some measure of competence.

After thirty-three years of getting my own way with more than I care to reiterate, I came to the end of my rope and was ready to leave everything to find something. I wanted to come back to TLC. Besides not having any money, my brother pointed out that I just wanted to go there because it felt comfortable . . . he was so right.

So I looked for another place and gave away most of what I owned. At this point I had given up the idea that TLC was even an option. It was by chance, or so I thought, that I ended up on the phone with the director, Joel Sheets. He asked me how I was, and I told him it was all coming undone. He had me here in less than forty eight hours. God's word says that He calls us to Him. He's been calling me for decades . . .

This time was so different. I had a better appreciation for the opportunities offered me here at TLC. Early on I decided that seeking God had to be a priority. I laid everything else aside and started reading the Bible. I found God right where He had been waiting for me. By the third or fourth month I was trying to figure out how to hear from God. I made discovery after discovery, thinking I was getting so far, but in truth I was taking one baby step at a time. By the latter part of the second year, I began to understand the slow but steady progress I was making. With each break through I began to realize the scope of this journey. (However, I wish I had paid better attention to my physical well being. I have managed to put on about a hundred pounds, but with the help of some friends, I am working on that.) I am glad that I spent the time the way I did. If I had worried about my appearance, as Solomon said in Proverbs, "Vanity, Vanity, all is vanity." I'm glad I didn't go down that road!

My wife has moved on. She is going through her own trials and well I can hardly blame her for not wanting to follow me into yet another era of my life. She has no reason to believe that it will turn out any different than any other time I tried to change. I continue to pray for her, and I hope that she is able to reconnect with God and find what I have found in Him.

I have spent much more time in my own head than with anyone else. It is a minefield. I have created more difficulties. I was so arrogant; I would have conversations in my own head and hold people accountable for the outcome. The negative became so prevalent that I was a total cynic. My perceptions, perspectives, and beliefs were so misguided that I was my own worst enemy; I didn't need any help. I tore apart my own life.

I spent the better part of my life believing I was a man of principle and high standards. I would put those standards on others and tear them down when they couldn't live up to them. I was so critical of everyone and everything. I thought I was some higher form of life. All I really had been was a man of high expectations—dumb enough not to understand why I was always let down. I wanted my dreams to come true, but I wanted to invest nothing in bringing them about.

I see it this way—don't spend time building every personal aspect of your own life and then put what's left over into your relationships. Truth be told, there is not likely to be much left if anything. If we don't put love and relationships first, than what will it matter what we have achieved or accomplished? Riches should be defined by the love and relationships in your life. What else could be so important?

I now have a relationship with my God; He has set me free from so many things. I've had to cry, mourn, wait, listen, work, surrender, and subject myself to God's will.

There have been trials and tribulations and I have had to persevere, but as a pastor of mine said, "God has not forgotten me, He sees me through and He keeps His word." He has kept every promise He has given me, and He is developing me into the man He created me to be. God is not finished with me; in fact He has only just begun. Yet, I have never been more at peace with the world in my life. There is a song "How He Loves" that has a line that says, "I don't have time to maintain these regrets, when I think of the way He loves me," that's where I am; I have more friendships, more peace, more joy, and more love for others than I have known in my life. There are those I miss, but God…

Life is so good, because God loves me so.

Broken Chains

Justin's Story

I was born in New Jersey and had two sisters. We lived with our mom, but I never met my real father. She remarried and we lived together until I was eight years old, and then she got separated because my stepfather was an alcoholic. My mom worked a lot after that, and we were left on our own—home alone. No one ever cooked for us. We basically grew up on the streets.

At age eleven I started drinking, then in middle school I started smoking pot. I dropped out of high school in my junior year. I was being hassled a lot by school counselors about my drug addiction. I was good with my hands and didn't care much about school anyway.

I went to work doing carpentry, landscaping, and general construction. I started doing heavy drugs—cocaine and sniffing heroin. I did it with friends here and there. I hung out a lot. My step dad died in 1996, and when he passed, I took a turn for the worst.

Drugs became a major priority. I got into a lot of fights. I was involved in gambling, poker games—that type of scene. In 2000 my mom died. I had nothing and no one to live for. Basically, I went to jail after that time until 2006. I was shooting heroin in prison.

In 2006 I went to the Good Shepherd Mission in Paterson. I ran into a friend of mine who was going there, and I went with him. By divine providence I was introduced to Jesus Christ, and I accepted him. I started working in ministries, singing in churches, getting to know God. I was in a program for eighteen months and graduated. I landed a union job while in the program, and I got my own place. I was working, going to Bible classes, and going to church. I stayed out of trouble for two months.

Then I was struck with a temptation to go out with a friend and shoot pool. I started shooting heroin again. My pride and bad attitude was coming back—my old way of thinking. I ran the streets for three weeks while working. I made a phone call to someone in the church and he called Transformation Life Center for me. He got a bed for me. I went through detox for four days before I came to TLC.

I came to TLC in December and repented of my attitude. Since being here my relationship with God is more real. I'm slowing down, not rushing through things. I'm developing a servant's heart, and understanding the significance of loving others and having relationships.

One major thing that's happened is receiving God's forgiveness, and putting into practice forgiving others. Things beyond my control happened to me in my childhood, and I had to forgive those people. I did a lot of counseling with a medic from the Bruderhof and also a lot of journaling. It allows me to express my feelings, to talk to God, and write down my thoughts and my prayers.

TLC has helped me a lot. It's different than other places, especially the relationships between the men. God's presence is also very real and very strong. You can feel him up here. I'm from Jersey and now I'm living on a mountain. It's great. You can take walks and look up at the stars and know He's there.

God has helped me to have self-control—one of the fruits of the Holy Spirit. I can now examine why I'm angry and I see it's pointless. It's more of a reaction, a habit pattern. My anger was a defense mechanism. I got angry and tough as a boundary to keep people away.

I never understood God before or His ways. I'm leaning to now. One day I heard someone on the radio say, "The Spirit of God ignites the Word of God. Without the Spirit, you won't be able to understand God." It has stuck with me, and I think about that a lot.

I want to be the kind of Christian who isn't ashamed to share the gospel. There was a time during dorm prayer that I shared about this with such passion, but I was addressing the other guys. I thought they were ashamed to talk about Jesus, but later I realized it was actually for me. Ever since then, I've never been ashamed to share again.

After that day I went out on "tables" into the community, which is something TLC does to raise community awareness and funds. Each time I've shared the gospel and what Jesus has done for me.

For the future I'd like to stay for the Resident Assistant program and then go to school to get my mobile crane operators license, and get hooked up in their union. I'm still in the roofer's union. I also want to get involved in a ministry that fits me. Now I know it's important to be involved with church, not to just attend. But I'm waiting for God to open up a door for me.

My advice to other addicts is—you'll never be free from addiction without Jesus Christ. He has set me free. From all the years of being in prison my heart was hardened, and I was so cold to others, but now my heart has been softened. I have compassion. Before I didn't care about anyone, now I'm concerned. Before, I was very angry and always fighting. Now I deal with my anger through self-control.

Jesus has given me a new identity and purpose. I now have an understanding of what true life's about. That brings a lot of peace, and I don't need drugs or alcohol.

No Longer Alone

Brad's Story

My name is Brad; I'm a second phase resident, and I was born and raised in Grand Rapids, Michigan. Growing up you would have never thought that I would turn to heroin to numb the pain. I had a family people dream of, but it shows that addiction is an equal opportunity employer. My mother and father were strong Christians, and I went to a Christian school. All this didn't stop me from feeling like I was a freak; I reached out to other cliques and was rejected. This made me feel so insecure and unsure of who I was.

Because I blamed my parents for putting me in Christian school, I started to rebel against them. Anything they asked I did the opposite to get their attention. I often did it to spite him. I blamed my problems on them. I didn't make friends in the Christian school, which became a big issue. I tried even more desperately to fit in time after time. In spite of my efforts to mesh with others, I was pushed to the edge of the crowd. Without anyone reaching out to me and teaching me, I was on my own to figure out who I was. I became depressed and suicidal. I'd cry in my room and started cutting myself to relieve the mental pain.

I went to counseling, and the psychiatrist put me on antidepressants. I was diagnosed bipolar, manic, and possibly schizophrenic. I went for nine years of Christian counseling, but it didn't help at all. It made me realize my problems, but they gave me no way to deal with them. They diagnosed me with a disease, which was counterproductive. They never talked to me about God. They were more into the secular philosophy of taking medication. I didn't want to hear it. This was darkest time of my life. I went through a long period of loneliness. I had no friends. I was cutting myself and hearing voices—you're worthless, kill yourself. It was strange because no one in the family suffered from depression. No one understood it.

In ninth grade, I dated a girl who lived down the street from me. She became everything to me. I finally got affirmation from a woman, my girlfriend. The love we shared was shallow and eventually I found out she was cheating on me. I grabbed a hunting knife and tried to cut my hand off at the wrist, trying to kill myself. (I still have a nasty scar.) The cops showed up, and I was angry that I didn't die. The pain was so great. I was in such confusion; I wanted to die—nothing mattered. I felt like my world's bottom had fallen out. I made a conscious decision, since I couldn't kill myself right, I was going to do as many drugs as I could and enjoy a slow death. Reaching out to coke, weed, acid, and heroin turned ugly quickly.

I was led into doing heroin from people I knew. I started working full time to support my habit. I had nothing to my name. I moved out of my parent's house by eighteen. I blamed them for all my problems. I wanted to be kicked out, living on my own. I went to rehabs and secular detox programs for twenty-eight days. I never would stay clean. I had a lot of partying friends at this time and was dating another girl. She thought she could help me, but then she left me. I was twenty-three when she left. I tried to commit suicide again.

All this time, I was still close to my mom, but there was an underlying tension with my dad. I didn't know what to do, so I moved back home. I was staying there until I could figure out what to do. One day I ran into a friend of my dad's who works for Set Free Ministries. I went out to lunch with my dad and this guy happened to be there.

He noticed I had cuts on my arms, and he said "Looks like you're hurting. Did you rebel? Rebellion is as the sin of witchcraft" (1Samuel 15:21). The amazing thing is I kept listening to him and he continued. "God has set his face against those who have practiced witchcraft. People used to cut themselves as a form of worshipping Satan." This reaffirmed the darkness in my life. He asked, "Did you not honor your father and mother? This is the first commandment with a promise—are your days going well? If you want to talk, here's my card." His words and those scriptures cut me to the heart.

Those few sentences told me more about my problems than nine years of counseling. God's word illuminated inside of me. It made so much sense. I called him after three days and talked to him. He explained my need for a Savior. I accepted Christ; I had never made the personal choice to accept Jesus. For the next nine months we studied the Bible and examined different sins. I confessed and renounced false beliefs, witchcraft, sexual sins, anger etc. I became so free. I quit using drugs. Then the doctor put me on Suboxone, which is a partial opiate and easier to get off of than heroin. You can control it. It worked well to get rid of withdrawals, but I was on this for two years.

I started a handy man business, and I was growing in my faith, but I was still depending on a substance. When the doctor took me off, I went back to heroin. I went back to cocaine, also, shooting everyday for a year. I was going to church, but I'd have to get high before I'd go, just to maintain, to be normal and at least function, so I wouldn't be sick from the withdrawal.

I thought I didn't need help, until God got my attention with three felonies, and a four-to-eight year prison sentence, all within a couple of months. I was also on probation for cocaine use and got caught with heroin. I was facing three felonies, carrying a minimum of eight years. My lawyer said I needed to get into a program, and then the judge might work with me. Four months ago my aunt told me of a guy who went through the Transformation Life Center program thirteen years prior, and she asked if I would be willing to meet with him. I didn't want to do anything about it yet, but then God brought this situation into my life to help me make the decision to come in January of 2009.

As soon as I got to TLC, I knew I needed to be here. I had a positive attitude. In the first couple of weeks I made friends and was applying what I was learning. I was changing and feeling God's presence as well as His peace and joy. The first six months impacted me so greatly. Since I've been at Transformation Life Center, the Lord has given me a vision and a future, but not before he dealt with my "heart condition." I still had a lot of insecurities and a fear of other people. Dope had numbed the voices in my mind telling me I wasn't good enough, that everyone was better than I was. I had to overcome those types of thoughts through Christ.

In the first six months, I had only scratched the surface, and I wanted to learn more. I've decided to stay for the Resident Assistant program. I want TLC to be a training ground for the rest of my life—teaching me how to be in ministry and the huge importance of fellowship. I was good at secluding myself, but it's so important to stay connected. I'm learning about myself and TLC is training me to help others, and giving me the desire to serve God.

TLC has helped me to learn how to apply God's word. My problem wasn't drugs, but a "heart condition." They helped me seek God for guidance, and purpose in life and now my life has meaning. I'm precious to God. He has great things planned for me. I want to stay at TLC until I hear different—until I've learned how to work with people, how to fundraise, and counsel others as well as receive counsel, and be a leader. I know God has a place in ministry for me. I'm content being here and no matter where He has me go, I'll have peace and joy. He'll put me where He can use me the most.

I want to go out and serve the Lord in ministry. I plan on spending my free time as a youth group leader. I want to let kids know that drugs aren't the way to get affirmation. I pray that God will open the door for me to speak to an audience about disobedience and the pitfalls that can result. I want to live a life in pursuit of righteousness, and I want to encourage others through my testimony.

I want to say to other teens—it's important to pick your friends wisely, choose to make friends, be involved. It's easy to hide the pain, be honest and open. You need the strength of Christ to do this. You can't be free of depression and have true joy without Christ. That empty hole can only be filled with Christ.

To parents I say—I took my frustration out on my parents. I knew they would still love me. Don't give up. Keep praying. My parents prayed for twelve years for me. Things kept getting worse until I finally hit rock bottom, but they didn't stop praying. Let your kids know you love them, but don't interfere. The more my parents tried to help, the worse it got. I did more to hurt them. It's important to give kids their space. You need to have tough love. My mom would often step in, but finally she made the choice to be tough. She let me stay in jail, which was a wake-up call. Things had to get so bad to the point where I had enough. And it did. I accepted Christ as my Savior.

God is No Longer Greek to Me
George's Story

I was born in Chicago in the 1960's to a Greek family. As a baby, I had bad allergies and wasn't doing well physically. Our doctor suggested we move to a dry climate, but my parents didn't have the money, so they sent me to Greece to live with my grandparents. I got better, but after six months they had lost a lot of their money in the stock market and were having problems. I stayed in Athens, Greece until I was five. I was spoiled by grandparents; they did everything for me.

When I returned to America I went to kindergarten without knowing how to speak English. It was difficult there in Chicago for me, and I learned at an early age how to defend myself in school. I grew up in a rough neighborhood and was a big, husky boy.

At the age of twelve I tried my first cigarette, at thirteen, my first beer, and at fourteen—drugs. My life consisted of going to parties and clubs while dealing cocaine in the neighborhood where I was employed. Later, I worked in the Chicago stock market and also dealt drugs there to the stockbrokers. I was selling cocaine to someone every night, but one night this one guy wanted a lot more than usual, and I turned him down. He got busted. He was trying to set me up.

I was told by my boss that I needed to leave; I was being implicated in selling drugs. The other broker got caught, but I got fired. So I went to Florida for a year and was introduced to crack because cocaine was scarce. People use to think I was a cop because I use to have to go to the ghetto to get my drugs. Then, I came back to Chicago and stayed clean from cocaine. I didn't hang out with the same crowd, but I did other drugs. In 2000 I overdosed on cocaine, but I didn't know it. I passed out for three days. When I went to the doctor, he told me I had overdosed. My family started looking for places for me to go, but everything was much too expensive. I was still snorting coke as they looked for a rehab.

One day I was working at the Greek restaurant my father managed, and I began to feel desperate over my situation with my addiction. I grew up Greek Orthodox, and knew little about God and even less about Jesus, but I said a simple prayer—"If you're there God and still listening, have mercy on me and my mother."

My mom had found out about Transformation Life Center from our family doctor, and he recommended I go there. I ended up in TLC in December of 2001 and stayed for a year. In 2002, I relapsed and came back and stayed for another year. I did nine months as staff doing whatever I was asked. I also helped implement the second phase— Resident Assistant. I put some structure into it. After working there, I decided to go to Bible College. I had a Bachelor's degree, but I had paid others to get it. Now I wanted to study the Bible.

The Bible clicked with me. The New American Standard Bible is the same as the Greek Orthodox Bible, but its simple language was never spoken in our church when I was growing up. It was always in an ancient tongue. When I go back to the neighborhood, I claim to be a Greek Orthodox Christian. I tell them they don't even know what the Bible says. I ask them, "Have you ever picked up the Bible?" All of my family is now saved; my mom came to know the Lord through Tom Mahairas, the founder of Transformation Life Center. My dad now loves the Bible and is in the Word of God a lot.

After I graduated from Bible College, I was praying about what to do next. I had pursued a four year education at Davis College and received a Bachelor of Arts in theology and counseling. Then I went on to get my Masters at Philadelphia Bible University. I also met my wife in undergraduate school and got married in 2006 to Angela. We've been married for three years. When I called TLC to congratulate the new director there, Joel, about his promotion at TLC, we talked about what I was doing. I needed to do twenty hours a week as an intern in counseling. He offered me a fulltime staff position along with the internship, so I came here with my wife, and I'm doing both.

It's fitting for me to return to TLC, as I was saved here. I didn't know the Lord before. After my first three weeks there, I opened up the Bible for the first time and read Psalm 40: 1-3:

> I waited patiently for the LORD; And He inclined to me, And heard my cry. He also brought me up out of a horrible pit, Out of the miry clay, And set my feet upon a rock...He has put a new song in my mouth— Praise to our God; Many will see it and fear, And will trust in the Lord.

All those years I was crying out for help. He heard my one prayer and took me out of Chicago, and set my foot on a rock at Transformation Life Center. My old identity was a junkie. My new identity is as a child of God.

TLC gave me the foundation of my Christianity. I've now been in Bible school for six years. What I learned at TLC, I didn't see out there in the world, however, I know we are still human and have faults.TLC helped me understand that and recognized my need to be a man—being addicted kept me a teenager.TLC helped me get in touch with my desire to be a man, to have a family, get married, and be a husband, and admit I have feelings. Before, I couldn't say I've been hurt. But the Lord put those emotions in us, so I can be a man and still admit to having feelings.

I had turned to drugs because I was missing my parents. Coming from Greece, I was spoiled by my grandparents, and I had needed to be disciplined. My mother's discipline shocked me, shattered me, and even crushed me. I felt like nothing was good enough, even though I needed the discipline.

In addition, coming from that rough neighborhood and being jumped all the time, made me tough. At twelve I made a conscious determination that no one was going to hurt me. Up until I was thirty-one, I kept that philosophy. I also thought that my mom and dad hated me, which was the furthest thing from the truth. Now, our relationship has been renewed. I went to Chicago and stayed with them for the first time in ten years. God has restored all things, and He can do it for you.

Once you accept that your addiction has taken over your life, only then are you on your way to recovery. My new normal is… not drinking, not working where I worked before, not hanging around the same people or places. By doing that I was able to be free of addiction with God's help. At first, while at TLC, I thought maybe I could go back and get a Bible certificate. God made me go much further.

My real goal was to get a Master's degree in counseling, which I will now have. I wanted to give back to the drug addiction ministry. The Lord put that on my heart. It's my passion to give back.

In May of 2010, I'll get my graduate degree, and then I will pursue a doctorate in strategic leadership at Regent University. I want to be in an upper management position in a Christian drug rehab. With God's help, I will.

Change of Heart

Jeremy's Story

I came from a good family and went to Catholic school, but I never had a relationship with God. When I was seven years old my mother got divorced. This gave me a lot of free time to get in trouble. I started smoking pot in eighth grade, and a few months later I started selling it. Although I was involved in sports in junior high and high school, I didn't hang around with those kids. I disliked Catholic school and as soon as the day was over, I went straight to see my friends in public school. I got in with the skater crowd and loved it. Skateboarding was my passion.

I continued selling pot and smoking it until I was sixteen, then I started using LSD. One day I stayed up all night and watched as the people came out of their houses and went to work. They seemed like herds of cattle, being controlled by society, and I never wanted to do that.

When I was seventeen, I moved to Ithaca with my mother. At first I didn't like it, but then she let me go to public school, and I was thrilled. Unfortunately, I got in with the wrong crowd and never graduated. By age eighteen, I started doing heroin and other opiates with them. After a while, I wanted to get clean so I went to Maui. I stayed there and got a job in a tropical flower farm, which I really liked. I got clean from opiates, but I started drinking alcohol every day. I stayed in Maui for six months, but I missed my old friends, so I moved back to Ithaca. Sometimes I lived with my mom and at other times with friends.

I got heavily into selling massive amounts of marijuana and moved up the ladder quickly. I made a lot of money. By the time I was twenty, dealing drugs took over my life. By twenty-three I had made enough money, and I felt I was ready to retire.

I moved to Colorado and rented a mansion in the mountains. I had everything you could want—cars, motorcycles, and a beautiful house. I set up a few people in the business, and was doing well, making a lot of money, but I was still drinking every day, and doing meth and cocaine. I blew through my money quickly, and I wanted to get clean from the hard drugs. I decided to visit a friend in Oregon.

On the way there, I totaled my car and was arrested for DWI. My landlord seized everything I owned and kept it all. I had a whole marijuana production plant going on inside the house, and I lost everything. I became really depressed and couldn't get back up. I felt I had nothing going for me—I hadn't even graduated high school, and I kept spiraling downward.

I moved back to Ithaca and really started to lose it. I started injecting drugs with needles when I said that I would never do that, but I didn't care anymore. I felt my life was done and there was no starting over. What did it matter anyway? Everything I had worked for was gone. I had neglected my education and had failed at everything. At twenty-three years old I felt hopeless, but I continued in that life style for another year.

One day in desperation, my mother dragged me out of where I was staying and took me to the hospital. I talked my way out of rehab and continued on the same course for six more months until my twenty-fifth birthday. My whole family confronted me, and I finally went to a twenty-eight day secular program and did well. I moved to New York City to Bedford Stuyvesant and was on a prescription drug that I was supposed to stay on for two years, but my insurance ran out. I had kept the name of one of the guys I met in rehab who lived in the area, and he hooked me up with the dope I needed. I was off to the races. I had two jobs, but was doing drugs again. I was a functional addict, until I couldn't hold down the jobs anymore, and I was fired. I spiraled even further downward.

One day I knew I had had enough, and so I reached out to my family. My mom had given me the phone number of a guy from church, Owen Kelly. I had held onto it for a year, but I finally called him. He recommended I go to Transformation Life Center. I went to my father's to detox and then came to TLC.

I am incredibly grateful that I came to TLC. From day one it was awesome. Everyone was so friendly, kind, and welcoming from the day I set my foot on campus. I accepted the Lord within the first month. I had been exposed to Christianity through my mother and my aunt, but I never had a relationship with Jesus. My grandmother was a devout Christian and she had been praying for me a lot. I now have found Christ and now live in faith serving at TLC.

TLC had done so much for me. First, it's the longest I've been sober since I was fourteen. Second, it has given me hope for a new life and a future. Third, I have a peace I never had before. Next, God has taken away my fear of the future, and last, I can trust God to provide.

I'd like to close by saying to anyone else going though an addiction that I know you can be a new creation in Christ. There is hope for a future for you and a better life. Don't believe the lie that once a junkie, always a junkie. God can do the impossible. He did it in my life.

Coming Back to Life
Ray's Story

I was born in Little Ferry, New Jersey. Growing up was rough. I was verbally and physically abused by my father who had a drinking problem, which only got worse after his mom died. This went on for several years, and the only thing that he ever said to me was, "You know I love you and I would never hurt you." The abuse and my dad's drinking were never talked about. I had low self worth, and I never thought I was good enough. I thought abuse equaled love, which destroyed many of my relationships.

I started using drugs when I was twelve. When I was thirteen, we moved to West Milford, NJ. My mom did this because she thought things would change. It was a nice thought, but it didn't work out like she had hoped. Things went well for a little while, but about a year later the hell started all over again and eventually my dad left.

From here on, my life was centered on using drugs and messing up relationships. I even lost two jobs because of my drug use. After going to a detox one year, I got a job with my uncle and did well for a while, but I felt empty inside. I was still getting high after work, and eventually on the way to work. This quickly got out of hand and my uncle fired me. I got upset with him. I was lost, scared and had nowhere to turn. I started doing more drugs—cocaine and oxycontin.

Then I lost one of my best friends to a drug overdose, which took me to new lows in my addiction. You would think that something like that would stop me from using and help me realize how serious this all was, but I only cared about myself. I thought I was the only one being hurt. I was wrong; my friends and family were watching me slowly kill myself. My mom always cared about me, even when I gave up on myself. She always had hope.

One day I stole my mother's car and drove to Paterson, N.J. I dropped the car off, but I didn't come home for two days. I was crying out for God's help, but I didn't know what to do. My mom was really upset, and when I came home, she drove me to a detox for three days. After that, they sent me to a thirty-day hospital program. I didn't want to be there. I complained a lot. I wanted my mom to come get me, but she wouldn't pick me up. They put me in a MICA unit. I was on five different medications for: bipolar disorder, ADHD, depression, anxiety, and a sleeping disorder. I told them it helped me, and that I was fine, so they discharged me.

My mom picked me up. I felt shot down because she was upset over everything. Within a half an hour of coming home, I used some birthday money to get high on heroin. I went right back to doing what I was doing before, but more discreet. I stole my mom's jewelry and pawned it. She didn't know about it. She thought I was doing okay, but I wasn't.

A few weeks later my mother came over to my place to give me a ride. While we were driving in the car, she got a call from on intake counselor at a rehab—Transformation Life Center. My mom asked me to talk him, so I did. I was broken and beat down by the world, so I was willing to listen to Erik, never knowing that God would use him to save my life. I could tell by his voice that he really cared. He asked me something like, "Can you keep doing what you are doing?" That question made me think.

I had tried a couple of rehabs before, but only to please everyone else. I hadn't wanted to stop using drugs because I didn't want to face all of the day-to-day struggles and all of my past hurts. I wasn't ready. But then something changed. I figured that going to TLC couldn't be any worse than the life I was living. In some ways it was a relief that I couldn't keep doing what I was doing.

The next thing I knew I was at TLC learning about God and gaining a new life. My relationship with my dad is being restored, and I believe he is even slowly coming to God. When I first got to TLC I was diagnosed with Lyme

Meningitis. I am grateful that God brought me here when he did, or I might not be alive today. Praise God for men like the ones at TLC who have a servant's heart and the love of Christ.

This program is different than any other I've experienced. It's not like other rehabs where everyone is talking about drugs and trying to outdo each other with their stories. I like TLC because we get through to the underlying issues. We deal with the deep stuff, not just the surface problems. We talk about our struggles and issues, which helps to reveal our real problems. Mine was my bitterness towards my father because he beat me. I had such low self-worth. I was also a people pleaser. I didn't like to say "No" to other people. I thought so poorly of myself, and I had problems forgiving my father. All of that is changing now.

My greatest success has been graduating from the six-month program, not just for the personal gain, but for everything—knowing God, my physical, mental and spiritual well being, the mended relationships, and the joy and peace. TLC has opened so many doors for me and has given me hope. It has changed my life.

Because of what has happened since being at TLC, my priorities have taken an about face. Number one is my relationship with God. I now spend time reading the Bible, praying, and asking Him for help. I know he cares for me. My family has become really important, especially my mom. I never use to hang out with her, but she's been great. We spend time talking about deep things and feelings. The whole atmosphere in the house has changed for the better. It's peaceful. I even have a healthy relationship with my dad.

I know some of you parents might be worried about your kids. Pray for them; don't plead with them. I know I didn't want to stop, so it didn't matter what my parents said or did. I admitted I had a problem, but I didn't want to change. I had to hit rock bottom. But that doesn't mean you should give up on them, keep praying.

I'm so grateful to God and for TLC. It's shown me how to live right. It's given me a new outlook on life—an eternal future.

The Simple Truth

Erik's Story

You can't always tell by someone's background what kind of choices they will make. I lived what most thought was a normal life. I am the oldest of three, with one brother and one sister. When I was young we did a lot of family activities and vacations, but as I got older I remember my father pulling further and further away, often with the explanation of a headache or other plans. My mom was the one who made sure that the three kids attended church every Sunday, but I honestly can't remember my father ever setting foot in the church. By the age of twelve I knew something wasn't good between my parents, and by the time I was seventeen, my father sat me down with my mother and told me that my they were getting divorced. I handled it like I handled everything else, acting as if it didn't matter or bother me.

I attended Rutgers College, but because of finances and the fact that it was close enough to my house, I commuted. I was not very active in the school party scene, but I did start hanging out with friends from the restaurant where I was working. I experimented with marijuana at the age of twenty-one, but I was never really into it. I completed school and continued to work in restaurants, where I met a girl that I started dating, and later got engaged to. Our relationship quickly went downhill after the engagement though, and we broke up. While we were apart she got pregnant, and when I found out about it I offered to raise the child with her, so we got married.

After my son was born, he was diagnosed with a syndrome called RTS, which causes significant delays in speech, coordination, and most other aspects of life. With the attention required by a special needs child, the already shaky marriage got worse. She started to hang out with old friends, and drugs soon followed. With the strain of everything going on, I began to use cocaine with her. Before the drug use could get too bad, she became pregnant again, and our party scene was temporarily put on hold. But after my daughter's birth, we both started using cocaine again. By the age of twenty-nine I was introduced to heroin. She started to inject it, and I soon did too. It all went downhill from there.

I lost my home, my career, my vehicles, and my children were taken away. I blamed everyone else for what happened. I continued in this lifestyle and wound up arrested. That was when the family found out about my drug use. I thought I would quit, but after several methadone clinics later, I was still using as much as ever.

I finally went to a twenty-one day rehab. I was hoping for a quick-fix answer to a much deeper problem, and after about sixty days I found myself back into drugs.

Two arrests later I wound up back in jail in Bergen County. Nobody would bail me out unless I came to a long-term program called Transformation Life Center. So in August of 2006 I agreed. The atmosphere at TLC was very different than anywhere else. I was given the opportunity to understand the gospel message, and how it applied specifically to me. I thought that I had come to TLC to address my heroin addiction, but I found out what I really needed was to allow Christ to heal the wounds of my childhood that I had been avoiding with the substance abuse. When I identified what was going on inside of me, I was able to let Christ work in me.

TLC has impacted my life and given me a greater understanding of relationships and family values. I can now forgive myself for the mistakes I've made which led to my greatest failure, the loss of my children. To date, I do not have communication with them, but I am learning to be patient for when they come back into my life.

Early in the program, a divorce from my first wife was finalized. But God replaced an unhealthy marriage with a new, Christ-centered one. I met Lisa, then a staff member at a Christian program for women similar to TLC, while giving my testimony. We began dating, and as of September 2008, we became husband and wife. Lisa had a daughter who she saw on weekend visits that she introduced into my life. I now get to spend time with my stepdaughter, who is about the same age as my son. I am grateful that God has entrusted me with this beautiful family.

After getting married Lisa came to TLC, and we now have the opportunity to work in ministry together. She works as the development coordinator, working with a team to provide support to the ministry in many important ways. I am the program coordinator at TLC, facilitating different areas such as the advisory team, classroom scheduling, teaching, and intake.

My advice to men and women with life-controlling issues is to learn from my mistakes. I'm thirty-six and I feel like I'm just getting started in life, but at least I learned my lesson. "An intelligent man learns from his mistakes. A wise man learns from other peoples mistakes." It is never the substance, but rather the lifestyle, and the spiritual and emotional wounds that go unaddressed.

Since coming to TLC, my priorities have changed drastically. My first priority is my relationship with God. I'm trying to always respond in a Christ-like manner. I want to be a loving husband to my wife and a good example to my stepdaughter. I also want to be available to others. What I'm doing is less important. My relationship with my family has become very important. I'm on good terms with my mom, and I see her frequently. My relationship with my dad, which had always been shaky, has become healthy and we talk often.

We're all trying to work together here at TLC to form a united front in "Transforming Men to Transform the World," with the help of Jesus Christ. I'm glad to have returned to His truth and to worship Him, instead of the things of this world.

From the Streets to God's Arms

Jesse's Story

I grew up on the streets of New York City. My life started going downhill at the age of eleven. With the help of my cousin, I was selling marijuana to make money, and I really enjoyed the lifestyle. I wanted to be my own boss and start selling drugs on my own. I wasn't brought up with a spiritual background or any form of church in my life, but I started attending church in 2003. At this time, my mom was going to kick me out of the house, and I felt as though I had no other option. Although no one in my family was a Christian, I thought I could play the "God-game" and make my family happy.

I was drawn to the pastor, and although I caused trouble, he showed me kindness. This pastor involved me with Christian music, which I really enjoyed. However, just as I had begun to form a meaningful, spiritual relationship with him, circumstances changed and he had to move to New Jersey. I remember becoming increasingly angry and felt as though I had no support; I questioned myself as to why I had tried to escape from my former life style. I began drinking and smoked marijuana heavily. I then tried smoking crack and quickly became addicted.

I had heard of a Christian camp in New York State called Citi-Vision that helped inner-city kids to form a relationship with Jesus Christ. I attended this camp for a summer to check it out, but I gave the staff there a lot of problems, as I rebelled against their rules. I managed to deceive the staff and would find ways to use drugs while I was there because I was addicted.

I remember that I was always so quick to attack and defend myself when I felt like someone was correcting me or even trying to get close to me. My anger made me realize that I had a problem, but I moved back to the city regardless, because I knew that that was where I could get more drugs.

At this time, I had lost a lot of friends and family from the chaos of the streets, so I decided to move back to Citi-Vision. Once there, I continued to play my game of heavy drinking and drugging. One day I came very close to death from all of the drugs in my system. I was so distraught that I was unsure whether to seek out help for myself, or more importantly, if I really had enough self-worth to even bother.

The next day Citi-Vision helped me make a call to a Christian rehab, Transformation Life Center. The staff interviewed me and was of the opinion that I was real bad news and would not adapt well there. Thank God the

Director, Joel Sheets, fought for me. My first week at TLC, I began to notice something very different from anything else I had seen before. The men at TLC had a peace about them as they praised God, yet I realized that all of this was taking place in the midst of turmoil in their lives. I became spiritually broken and humbled, watching them and wondering if I could also share this experience. I tried following as they did, but nothing changed for me. I had some knowledge of God, but I didn't know very much.

Then one night, I walked outside on my own and prayed to God that He would come into my life. I prayed, "God, if You are real, please come into my life because I know You love me. Change me, teach me, and show me what to do." I didn't feel anything that night or for the next three months. I also didn't receive any mail or hear from anyone I knew. Someone in the program told me that, "It's not about what you feel; but more often, about what you do."

One day, I just woke up and felt the greatest peace I had ever felt. Even when people would criticize and frustrate me, I felt it only natural to show love and help them, instead of continuing to hurt. I had a renewed love for God and a hunger for learning about Him, and I decided to enroll in the Word of Life Bible College. Some of the people in the college were harder to deal with than the men at TLC. I still managed to get through and finish school after a year of being molded and learning a great deal.

A while after I was out of the program, I thought I could give up on God and I *tried* to go back to the city and the drugs. It was not the same; I found no fulfillment in my actions. I did not find the happiness or pleasure that drugs used to bring. I continued using for several weeks and came to the realization that I had to remove myself from this environment.

By the mercy of God I was able to go back to CitiVision for another four months and again, involved myself with God. After the four months, I felt it right to move on. I made the decision to move to New Jersey and became deeply involved with a church, and I found a good job. God placed a desire within my heart to go into the pastoral field. I have been able to help out in my church by assisting with the youth groups, bringing new people to the church, going to school, and waking up early to get into God's Word to start off each day. God has changed my life dramatically. I found what I was looking for in His arms. His ways are awesome.

Starting a New Life

Mark's Story

My name is Mark William B.; I was born on March 26, 1989 at St. Anthony's Hospital in Warwick, NY. I was raised in a small town called Greenwood Lake and brought up in a Christian home. At the age of twelve I was baptized. My mother taught kindergarten at a Christian school, and my father worked as a Foreman for OTIS elevator in New York City.

When I was fourteen years old my father had a seizure on a job, and he got rushed to the hospital where they found a tumor on his brain. They then did some tests and diagnosed him with level four, geoblastoma, brain cancer and gave him three months to live. When I heard that news, I didn't know what to do, so I resorted to smoking pot and drinking alcohol. I tried my first bag of cocaine at the age of fifteen.

When I was in high school my father became sicker and sicker, and I was more and more involved with drugs. I tried everything I could get my hands on to numb the pain and not have to deal with the reality of my father slowly slipping out of my life. When I was in tenth grade I experimented with more serious drugs such as oxycontins, ecstasy, all types of painkillers, and an abundance of

133

cocaine. I stayed on that binge until the beginning of my junior year of high school.

My father died two weeks after my seventeenth birthday on April 2nd 2006, and that is when I completely lost it. The night of his death, I went out and got drunk and high, then hooked up with as many girls as I could—just so I could get my mind off the fact that my father was no longer in my life. I had lost my best friend and the only person I trusted. I cut everyone out of my life, including God, and I stopped going to church.

From there on out I got more involved with drugs and started selling every drug and doing them all for the simple fact that I didn't want to face reality. I didn't want to let go of my father's death. At the beginning of my senior year, I ended up getting arrested and got kicked out of school for three months because it was drug and alcohol related. This ruined my high school and wrestling career.

During that three month period, I got heavy into cocaine and oxycontin, and I overdosed. I was clinically dead for five minutes. After that I got involved in heroin and crack cocaine, and I wanted nothing more than to die, which was my main goal.

In February of 2008, I got arrested and thrown into jail in Paterson, New Jersey for possession of seventeen bags of heroin. I got released on my own recognizance and went back home. I cleaned myself up for about a month until I heard my mother was getting remarried. I got mad at her for remarrying and I moved out and went back on the street.

I got more heavily involved in heroin and crack cocaine. I just didn't want to stop, and I started doubling everything I was doing just to get away from my pain and reality. I eventually got arrested and thrown back into jail on August 8, 2008. I spent about a week or so in jail, and my mother bailed me out on the condition that I go to Transformation Life Center.

I came up to TLC and spent six months as a resident. The program here gets down to the core issues of why you do drugs: mine were anger, resentment, mistrust, and depression. I'd been in an outpatient rehab before and went to that program high; it did nothing for me and I met people there just to buy drugs from them. Transformation Life Center is completely different. It has helped me turn around one hundred and eighty degrees. I planned on staying for only a month and have been here for over six.

I'm currently in the second phase doing another six months as a Resident Assistant. I have completely changed my life and have given it all up to God. I couldn't have made it through all this if it wasn't for Him looking out for me and making sure I didn't succeed at my goal of killing myself. I am now looking to go to college and make something out of my life. I want to make an impact on the lives of other people. I'm thinking about being a drug and alcohol counselor. I want to help other people, especially young people; I can relate to them.

My greatest success has been completing the first phase of this program. I never completed anything else before. My worst failure was my decision to do drugs and not caring what others thought. My uncaring attitude hurt those who loved me. My mom didn't really believe what was happening to me. She was in denial until I was put in jail.

My advice to parents is: don't be afraid to step in if you suspect something. Say something to your child. Talk to them and try to find out the problem. Get them some counseling if they're willing to go.

My advice to other addicts is—GET HELP. There's no reason to keep doing what you're doing. It's not doing anything good for you. There are other ways to deal with your issues. God is good, and He is definitely the way. He turned my life around, and He can turn yours around too.

I have a quote I made up that I live by now, "I have hurt many people in my past, and I have hurt myself, but now I'm a changed man, and I plan on making an impact whether you believe (that) or not."

Giving God a Chance

Stephen's Story

My name is Steve, and I was born and raised in New Jersey. I was adopted as a baby and have one brother. I had a great pair of parents and wanted for nothing. My mother was Catholic, and I had to go to church until I was fourteen. I believed in God, but I didn't have a personal relationship with Him. As I got older, I started hanging out with unpopular kids—the freaks and hippies. I never liked school. I didn't like sports, but my dad and brother did. My father tried to force me into little league, but I didn't like it. I just stopped going to practice.

I started experimenting with alcohol at a young age, stealing liquor from my parents who had it there for company. I did that on the weekends, but I never really liked alcohol. In the summer of sixth grade, I started smoking weed. In the early 70's, others accepted it, especially in my kind of work—construction. We would do lines of speed. This went on in my teen years, and I got more and more into drugs. I enjoyed drugs.

I also liked to work on things, trucks, cars, and machinery. My family is in the trucking and excavating business, so I spent time with my uncle and his machinery. Growing up as a kid, I would hang out with my grandpa

137

who taught me to work on cars. Mechanics was such a passion for me. I told my parents I wanted to drop out of school and work. I was a good mechanic. I worked on weekends with my uncle. When I went to high school for half day, I had a job working in a truck repair shop.

I got into trouble in school and was suspended for two weeks. My parents told me I had to make a choice—either go back to school or quit and go to work fulltime. I went back to school, but I told them I couldn't promise them I wouldn't get in trouble. My dad didn't want me to do construction work. But in eleventh grade, I quit school.

I started working full time at the trucking place, and I made more money so then I could buy more drugs. Then one day my boss confronted me. I couldn't come back to work being high all the time. I lost that job. I got a job as a laborer in a construction job, but I wound up being a mechanic there. At twenty, I got married and had two daughters. I was married for ten years, but I was a workaholic. I took after my parents with their business view. I was married to my job. I never came home. When we were together, we were doing a lot of drugs. One night I got into a physical fight with her. I left. I didn't want to beat her. We were growing apart, so we separated and then divorced.

My drug addiction got worse. I worked and partied all the time. Anything from acid to meth was the norm. Then I was introduced to heroin. That's when things started going downhill, fast. I did heroin for a year and a half. I lost job, my rights to see my kids, my apartment on the Jersey shore, my girlfriend—everything. I wound up on the street, but I was in jail most of the time.

On Dec. 27th 1999, my dad passed away. I went to his funeral in handcuffs and shackles. In March of 2000, my girlfriend overdosed and died while I was in jail. At that point, I gave up on life. I lived homeless for three and a half years, and wound up back in jail. After doing fourteen months I got out and called an old employer. He gave me a job. Two old friends of mine worked there—Sonny and Lamoure. They both knew the addiction lifestyle, but they had become Christians many years ago. They knew what Christ could do for me. I had no place to go, so I moved in with them.

I was going to an outpatient program while living with them. At the outpatient program, I got high. They told me I couldn't do that while living there. Sonny asked me, "What are you going to do with your life?" They told me about Transformation Life Center. I didn't want to go there. But they said, "You've tried everything else, see what happens." They had been witnesses to me—leaving me information, tracks, and cassettes for twenty years. I figured, okay; I'll try for a month. (I've now been here at TLC for over a year.)

Ten days after I came here, I gave my life to the Lord. I didn't know what to expect. I woke up one Saturday and everything was lifted—the guilt and the pain. I felt freedom. I started taking everything seriously. God has been good to me. It's such a better way of life. I stayed in the program for six months and graduated the first phase, but then I went out into the world. I had a job and was plugged into my church. I went to meetings and thought I was fellowshipping. I needed help, but I just told everyone I was fine. Since I didn't ask for help or seek godly counsel, I relapsed. After much persuasion by the director of TLC, I came back.

I recently finished the second phase of the program, being a Resident Assistant. It hasn't been an easy road for me. I prayed God would help me be a better father to my two daughters, but instead He gave me a camp of twenty-year-old men. I've recently been reunited with my daughters and love speaking to them every now and then. I've had opportunities to leave, but God wants me at TLC to be a spiritual father to these young men, to be still and listen, and see what God has in store for me. It's not what I want; it's what He wants.

The people at TLC are great. I never thought people would accept me so easily. God is doing amazing things. Being here and sharing with the guys how God has changed my life is healing me. I'm glad I don't have to go through the hell of being addicted anymore. Sure there was fun, but there is a high price to pay. The price is not worth it. Any suffering with Christ is worth it. True joy and freedom comes in Christ. I've stumbled a few times, but that's okay. I repent and God forgives. I can share that with the guys; I can go through trials. I get stubborn at times and bang heads, but God is teaching me.

When I spend time in the Word, God reveals to me that what we're doing here at TLC is important. I'm drawing closer to Him. What He teaches me with each trial prepares me for the next. As far as my future is concerned, I'm waiting to see what God has for me. I'm planning to stay at TLC until God changes my heart. They tell me I'm helping the guys here, though I don't see it. I try it keep the men in the program from falling or straying. I try to lift them up.

My advice to addicts is not to focus on the things of the world; Christ can change your life. Take this with all seriousness. It's your life you're dealing with. What do you have to lose? The streets will always be there. Give God a chance.

No More Destruction

Mike's Story

I grew up in Lodi, New Jersey with a good family. I was an only child and spoiled with affection. Though my parents were divorced when I was seven, I had a good relationship with them. I didn't have an absent father, but he wasn't present emotionally, even though he does love me. I started smoking weed when I was fourteen because I was looking for something else, something spiritual to view the world differently. I didn't experiment with any other drugs in high school.

I went to church up until I was seventeen, but once I got my car, I stopped attending church. After graduating from high school, I went to college for a year and worked at a pharmacy and started using oxycontin. That's how it all started. I did that for a year and then graduated from there to heroin. It's been a downhill ride ever since.

I had to keep hitting lower and lower bottoms. Every time I hit bottom, I continued with drugs because I thought I could find a successful way of using. It became my idol. I worshipped it in what I did, through my actions, and what I thought. I became homeless and was living in a cardboard box over the summer of 2005. I was still getting high. I had a girlfriend who was using also, and she enabled me. I had the bare minimum to survive, and that was all that mattered.

In the summer of 2007, I got clean from heroin and lived at home. Ever since then, up until summer of 2008, I'd cycle on and off drugs—using for a couple of months and then getting clean. I had a year clean off of heroin, and then I relapsed again in June of 2008. I realized I needed a long term residential program.

I had done twenty-eight day programs, hospitals, countless detoxes, Narcotics Anonymous meetings— nothing worked because I didn't participate. As soon as the meeting was over, I bounced. NA's focus is on physical sobriety, but there are many types of addictions that keep us in bondage, such as an addiction to sex. I needed more than what NA offered.

I heard about Transformation Life Center from my mother's nephew who graduated from this program, and she told me about it. At first I didn't want to go, six months was too much time. But after having burned so many bridges—quitting my job and dropping out of school, I had nothing else to do. I actually quit work and school on purpose so I wouldn't have any other options because I knew what the results would be if I continued to use heroin. I went through it enough times to know what happens. I wanted to back myself into a corner. I was at home for two months waiting to get into TLC. I wasn't getting high, but I was on a medication they give you at dextox. It was easy to be home, but I knew I needed to go to a program.

Finally, I got into the program, and I knew the struggle would begin. I went through a month of physical withdrawals. It was very uncomfortable the first couple of weeks. The first two months I was here, I was convinced I would only do three months. I didn't have any big breakthroughs. I already knew God because of the shelters I went to before. I started to know Him there. But then when I got here, I was trying to give myself the best chance of really recovering. I decided to stay so I could break the habit of not completing what I start. There were times I considered leaving, but I stayed because after all these years I understood myself—when I most wanted to leave is when I most needed to stay.

Here at TLC, I've learned to submit. I use to blow up when I was told to do something, but little by little I've learned to submit. I've used this as a real world exercise. There will be people in the world I don't get along with, so I'm trying to endure this. I really understand that ultimately God's in control. I'm trying to do what's right, as far as I understand it.

I've been here eight months and I'm in the second phase of the program as a Resident Assistant. I thought the RA program would be something very different than what it's turned out to be. I thought I was going to have a lot more time for myself and going home. Because of this, it's taught me patience. Sometimes things don't seem fair; I feel entitled to something better. But during these two months, I've been stretched a lot. I feel I've grown, especially after this one incident.

One Friday I was suppose to go home, but I hadn't handed in my homework. I was told I couldn't go home. Usually the punishment is applied after you get back, but not this time. So when I called home, they weren't fazed by it. I realized maybe it wasn't that big of a deal as I was making it. This incident helped me focus on myself, and what I need to do. I wanted to put the blame on someone else, but I finally came to grips with it after I calmed down. I came to the realization that if I would have handed in the homework on time, I would have been able to go. I learned an important lesson about consequences.

All the things that are in the world are here at TLC also, but that's good too. Here I've learned to deal with my emotions in a protected environment. I came here with a lot of Bible knowledge, but I was being a hypocrite. It's helped me learn not to react to things, to take a step back, see all the angles, and get a bigger perspective.

If I were a parent who suspected my child was doing drugs, my advice would be to talk to your child. Give them a drug test and educate yourself as much as you can about drug addiction. There's something else going on in their life. The addict doesn't realize what that is, especially at the beginning stages. Spend time with them and see if they'll talk to you about it. No one can make them stop; they have to want it for themselves, but you can help.

I hope my testimony will help other addicts. Take what you can out of it. Drugs are not worth the temporary high; they can destroy you. They aren't worth the consequences. Ultimately, drugs prevent you from facing your problems and responsibility. They create more problems that you need to deal with later on. The longer you're in the cycle, the harder it is to get out of it. You don't need drugs.

God is sufficient. His provisions are enough. I'm learning to believe that fully. I know my drug addiction has been terrible, but I know God works all things together for good. Now I know Jesus, and that is good. I could have had a normal life, but my spiritual eyes would have been closed. I wouldn't have seen the spiritual condition I was in, and for this I'm thankful.

Coming Home

Justin T.'s Story

I grew up in a Christian home and went to church every Sunday with my family. My parents were good Christians and didn't have a lot of struggles in the family. However, I never took church seriously. I never thought about the message. The stories from Sunday school seemed like fairy tales, so I goofed off in class and didn't pay much attention.

In school, I was quiet and reserved and felt very self-conscious. I didn't want to make others feel weird that I was a Christian, so I hung out with the misfits. I had some kind of social anxiety that I didn't understand at the time. I often skipped school with another friend of mine, so I didn't have to worry about being around a lot of people. I started smoking weed and it helped me focus. It slowed down my brain and I could be sociable. It made me feel accepted. I started finding those kids who were "pot heads." At that time I found a group of them, and I felt like I had friends for the first time. I felt as though I had come into my own. I had hated not having friends before. I justified smoking pot because it helped me socially.

I thought I would stop with just smoking marijuana, but I didn't. I started experimenting with other drugs like ecstasy and mushrooms. I skipped school a lot in my junior year, so they put me in a Christian school for the last half, even though they were having financial problems, and we were evicted from our home. There were a lot of new kids at the Christian high school, and I got in with the wrong crowd. I didn't want to be a Christian. I liked living in my sin. It was easier, and I didn't want to live upright, so I got pulled back into sin. A lot of kids got caught doing drugs, and I was kicked out of the school along with them. The rest of the year I was homeschooled, but I didn't pass.

In September, I went to high school at Newburgh Free Academy, which had a bad reputation. I did a lot of drugs and skipped school a lot. My parents were going through hard times, and we moved around a lot. We moved to New Windsor, and I dropped out of school. I moved in with my aunt because I was arguing with my parents. I wasn't with my friends anymore, so I started taking over the counter drugs. But then I moved out of her house, and I did drugs even more. I smoked pot every day, and then friends introduced me to cocaine. At first I started out doing it once in a while. I was living with a friend in an apartment, and I got my girlfriend pregnant. My mom wanted me to move back home, and I did—the day before my daughter was born.

I thought everything was going to be okay because I was going to be a dad. I was clean for two weeks. Then I started hanging out with my friends again. I went back down, but this time I went undercover. My girlfriend didn't know I was doing drugs, so about a year later we got married. We moved in with her parents. I was working two jobs—one at Sam's Club and another at Dairy Queen; I was a functioning addict. I was feeding my addiction more and more. I lied to her about why I was often in a bad mood and we argued constantly, but we moved in together into an apartment. One day she started going through my things and found my paraphernalia. I went on a three day binge of drugging. We had a lot of problems, and she started going out to bars. We tried going to counseling, but it didn't work. I wouldn't admit I was an addict. I left her.

I was gone for about eight months, living in my friend's basement, getting high, and always thinking about my daughter. Living like that gave me time to think about the destruction I was bringing. My family didn't know where I was. I was tired and wanted out of this. I could either call them or be homeless. I decided to call home and ask my mom what I should do. She said I should go to Transformation Life Center. I said "sure, why not." I was desperate.

When I first came to TLC, I felt I needed to be there once I met the guys. I cried when my parents dropped me off—six months seemed like forever. At first I went back into my shell. I wasn't comfortable. I started seeking God, and asked him why I was like this. My father was reserved. He backed up my mother, but was not the enforcer. But my brother was outgoing and friendly. I was jealous of him. I wanted to deal with this problem I had.

I found an understanding of who I was in the Bible. I started applying the things I learned in Sunday school to my life. My confidence wasn't in myself, but in God. God made me who I am. Now I enjoy praising God. I found a real energy inside of me. I started talking to others. This was new to me. I was open to everything—ready to receive.

Being at TLC, I've learned how to pray. I now have a relationship with God and my wife. Before TLC she wouldn't let me see our daughter, but now she has agreed. Before TLC she wouldn't give me the time of day. Now she will talk to me. Because of TLC, I have a deep joy that depends on God.

If you are a parent with teenagers, and you want to keep them away from drugs, my suggestion is that when you have to say "no" to something, explain why. Discuss why something is wrong and where such a path may eventually take them. Don't shelter them from your experiences. Be open minded and communicative so they will feel comfortable discussing issues with you. Be in prayer a lot.

If you are on the road to addiction or already addicted, there's nothing you can do to make yourself better. Only God can make you better; you can't do it within your own strength. I've tried, and it doesn't work. You need God's help. He's helped me a lot, and I'm truly happy with who I am for the first time.

A Time for Restoration

Scotty G.'s Story

I grew up in Hicksville, Long Island with two older brothers. We come from a privileged, middle-class background. My father was an electrician, but he had a lot of aggression, and there was a lot of yelling in the house when I was growing up. He didn't know how to discipline us three boys, and we were wild.

My drug and alcohol career began in my teen years. At first, I started drinking to fit in. My brothers and I started hanging out with friends in high school, which became one big party. Our parents were in the middle of getting a divorce, and they weren't aware of what was happening. Although I graduated, in my junior year I was arrested for assault, due to alcohol abuse. I got drunk and provoked a fight, so I spent time in jail. I had a job, but I was on probation because of my drinking.

On the weekends, I started smoking pot and drinking. I wound up cracking up my car and getting a DWI. I went to a twenty-eight day rehab just to satisfy the court. I was not trying to get clean. At that time, I was a functioning addict. From there I went to a halfway house in Arizona for seven months, but I wanted to get back to New York to see my girlfriend. I came back and went right back to the same lifestyle. After that, I went to jail for eight months.

I got saved in a jail cell in 1998. My brother Michael told me about Jesus. He had become a Pentecostal Christian. I got out of jail and rehab, and went right to church. It was a bumpy road. I kept going back and forth between drinking and being sober. I knew I was saved, but I couldn't give up the drinking.

At church, I met one of the board members of Transformation Life Center, Pat Clancy. He went to the same church I did, the New Hurley Baptist Church. He was leaving to go to TLC to be a full time board member, and he gave me a flyer. I was doing well at the time, but one of my brothers was doing poorly. He was involved with cocaine back in 2003-2004, so I took the information for him.

I spent a few years bouncing around from place to place, trying to be a Christian. Things fell apart for me, and I moved back in with my mother. I was doing a lot of coke at the time, and I knew I needed help. I decided to call TLC. They had a bed available for me, so I came up and went into the six-month program. I graduated in August 2007.

I realized a lot from that. I was determined to be a devout Christian, but my determination wasn't good enough. I went right back to using again. So I came back a year later. I'm now in the Restoration phase, and hope to be over and done with this problem. TLC has helped me so much. God allows you to come here through providential circumstances and gets you up here. It's an opportunity to be taken away from your environment and be introduced to Christ and a new way of life. You can see God's mercy at work to lift you out of the lifestyle you're in and to draw closer to Him.

I need to learn the truth, really learn it, and live it out to keep me from destroying myself. There's a big emphasis on application at TLC, putting what you learned into practice. You have to get down to where you struggle— your bad habits, undisciplined way of life, and doing what you want, and then overcoming it. Everyone who's addicted needs to embrace the struggle and not run away from it.

The first time around, I wanted to get out; I didn't want to be under the TLC authority. I wanted to be under the church authority. I was so self-centered and six months wasn't enough to get rid of that selfishness. I realized it was all about what I wanted—my wants, my needs, and not what God wanted. Now I've changed. I'm staying here at TLC until God opens the door for me to leave, and not before. I have no desire to go anywhere. I want to go where God wants me; He has been so merciful and kept me alive all these years.

If any of you reading this are parents and have a child struggling with an addiction, my advice to you is to get as many people praying as you can—that's where the biggest battle takes place, on your knees. Get in contact with TLC and let them know what's going on, ask them for prayer, and they will. Satan is very cunning, so you need to blow his cover and let others know about the situation so they can pray.

Though Satan enticed me, I take full responsibility for my choices, but I know God has worked things according to His plan. God has a particular saint struggling with a particular sin, so this saint can go to those people struggling with the same sin, and help them. I know I'm going to be okay now. I'm sick of being sick and willing to really change. God has finally gotten through to me. He's restoring my life.

In God's House

Steve's Story

A couple of years ago, I was sitting in my apartment drunk. I didn't need a reason for being in this condition; it's just the way I was. Anyway, I was sitting in my apartment because I was unemployed. I was unemployed because I was an alcoholic. My landlord had started eviction proceedings against me because I wasn't paying my rent. My power had been turned off by Central Hudson for non-payment of my bills. I was stealing power and cable from one of my neighbors. I was about to be kicked out of my apartment. I felt that I had nowhere to go or anyone to turn to, and then my father called me with an offer of help. It was an offer that was to completely change my life.

I didn't wake up one morning and decide to become an alcoholic. It was a process that took years to develop. Recognition of my drinking problem took even longer. I would blame negative happenings in my life on everything but drinking. It was always someone else's fault. I knew that was crazy thinking, but the consequences of facing the truth were too frightening. I lost jobs as a direct result of my drinking, but I would always blame the management for being biased against me for some reason or another.

When my wife and I divorced, I blamed her. I attributed all of our problems to her negative outlook of life. It's no wonder she had a negative outlook, she was married to a drunk. At one point, she told me to get help, and if I didn't I should pack my bags and leave. I told her that I didn't have any problems so I didn't need any help.

I ended up staying at my parents for a while. I eventually got a place of my own. It was a room in a rooming house. As cheap as that was I couldn't maintain the rent, and I ended up being kicked out of yet another place. At this time, I was still working so I was able to save up money for another apartment. I was okay for about three months then I started not paying my rent again. I was working just so that I could drink. I didn't care about anything else. My landlord had no other recourse except evicting me. He gave me all sorts of breaks, but I was such a jerk that I didn't see what he was trying to do for me. I was really feeling sorry for myself at this point in my life. I wasn't able to cope with everyday life without a drink in my hand. It was at this point that my father stepped in to rescue me from myself.

My dad had called me and asked me if he could come over and have a talk with me. I knew what it was going to be about, so I really didn't want him to come over. My apartment and I were in no shape for people to see us, but

I couldn't say no to my dad. When he arrived and we began to talk, he suggested I put myself in some kind of rehab program. By this time I knew I needed outside help. I simply couldn't keep going on like I was and expect to live much longer. I made the decision, with my father's help, to enter a rehab program. That decision has changed my life.

I entered into a six month long residential treatment program—Transformation Life Center. I ended up staying for eighteen months. It has been the best thing I have ever done for myself. While I was there, I recommitted my life to Jesus. When I did that, it opened up doors to me that had been shut and locked. I never thought I would be back in school, yet here I am taking an English class. I am now a member of my church. I am involved in the youth ministry at our church. These things were not possible for me a couple of years ago. Every day I wake up, I am amazed at the way my life has been changed.

My life has had its ups and downs, but due to the good decisions that I have made in the past two years and the actions of others, I hope to have many more ups than downs. I am no longer the self-destructive person I once was. Putting my drinking behind me and God in front of me has had many positive results in my life.

No Problem Too Big For God

Cody's Story

I was born in California, and I lived there with my parents until I was seven. My parents got divorced, and I got in trouble in school. I stabbed a teacher with a pencil. I recall being a very angry child, even before my parents got divorced. At the age of four, I started running away from home. I started hurting animals at a young age and started fires.

At age eight my step-father had a stroke, and he then died when I was ten. My mother got remarried when I was sixteen. I started drinking a lot then. My mother was an alcoholic, but she didn't know anything about my drug or alcohol abuse. I went to church to look good, and she thought I was okay. Though I was often in trouble in school, my grades were good.

We had moved to Arizona when I was eight. I loved the desert, but that didn't keep me from getting in trouble in school. I was always in a mess for one reason or another. I brought brass knuckles to school in seventh grade and got suspended the last quarter for getting into a fight. In eighth and ninth grade, I got in trouble for selling pills and weed. At sixteen, I moved back to California to live with my father.

I was diagnosed in school as being bipolar and schizophrenic. I was put on a lot of drugs—3,000mg of depacote, plus five other medications. I was doing okay, but I got back into selling prescription drugs. At seventeen, I had a bad trip on mushrooms. The cops came to my father's house and took me to the hospital. My dad found a quarter pound of weed, coke, and a scale, and he kicked me out. I moved back to Arizona.

Since I had survivor benefits from my step dad's death, I got my own house and lived on my own in a two bedroom house. I immediately got into selling drugs and started up my connections from when I was younger. I was smoking pot every day, working as a pizza delivery boy and snorting coke. I had two sets of friends—young ones who knew nothing about my older friends, with whom I was dealing drugs. I was also robbing a lot of houses and paying for my habit, selling stolen goods. Then my house got raided.

After my house was raided, my girlfriend broke up with me. I went into a tailspin. I was doing more drugs with a girl, Taylor, but I was trying to get in with this nice girl, named Emily. She was a Christian and wanted me to go to church with her, so I went. But I didn't stay long. I was high and I walked outside. Someone who could tell I was high, told me about Transformation Life Center. They gave me the number and I said I would call, but I didn't. I stayed up for a month doing drugs, then crashed and slept for four days. I finally called TLC and then went there.

At first I had a hard time because I was racist and there were nine black guys in the program. I had been hanging out with skin heads, and I was into white power. But after two months, I was saved and I started being less prejudiced. I became friends with one of the black guys. God showed me it didn't matter about skin color. Then I also had to deal with my anger. I almost got into some fights, but I was getting better, talking with people instead of fighting. I had to use self-control. I had no choice. I was stuck in the middle of the country in New York State. I had always been independent before, but now I see I don't need to be so dependent on myself.

I don't need to be alone all the time. I can depend on the body of Christ. Since coming to TLC and becoming a Christian, I'm not lonely anymore. I've matured a lot. I'm nineteen years old, and I've gained confidence in being me. My relationship with my mom has improved, and she's doing better with her recovery.

It will take me a year to graduate instead of six months because I got extra time for smoking cigarettes and drinking when I was going out in public—sitting at tables outside of business giving people information about the program. I've learned a lot from that. I was going to go into the military once I graduated, but now I've decided to stay six more months for the Resident Assistant program. God had more for me, and I had to surrender to Him. God can help me handle it.

When I graduate from the RA program, I plan on getting my high school diploma and going to trade school. After that I'd like to go into the Job Corps and then into the military, but for now I'm taking it one step at a time. I thank God for what He has done in my life. I forgive my brother for something he did that hurt me, and I pray for him every day. I hope we will be able to talk again and see each other soon, as the restraining order is ending soon. God has worked in me and changed my life for good.

Out of the Fire

Joe's Story

My name is Joe. I was born in Ridgewood, New Jersey, and I grew up and had a great childhood in Paramus, New Jersey. Through high school and college, I was never into the party scene. At age twenty-three, I got my dream job and was hired as a fireman. Two years later, I got married. It was the best day of my life.

Shortly after I was presented with cocaine, against my better judgment, I tried it. From that day on, I was hooked and began to make a series of bad decisions. Coke went to crack, and from there things got out of control. I started losing friends. I lost my job at the firehouse, and my wife left and took our newborn with her.

I went to a few secular rehabs just to please others. I wasn't ready to change. After getting arrested quite a few times, even once by a friend, I still didn't want to change.

One day I was on another run, and I had this urge to call my grandma. She, along with my Uncle Marvin, led me to TLC. I came to TLC with a lot of legal issues and as a last ditch effort to save my marriage.

Soon after I got to TLC, it became clear that I was living my life all wrong. I needed help because I just could not do it on my own. I accepted our Lord Jesus Christ into my heart and have not looked back. I have graduated from Phases one, two and three.

Through the year and a half at TLC, I have encountered many struggles, including a painful divorce. God has always been there to help me through all of these struggles. He has stood by me through my legal issues, and also gave me the privilege to watch Him transform other men's lives.

I have restored relationships with my father and other family members. This has meant so much to me. I also have a talking relationship with my ex-wife, and by the grace of God, I get visitation with my beautiful daughter Lauren.

God has transformed my life, and praise God for the work He is doing in transforming the lives of the other men at TLC.

Inner Peace and Joy

Austin's Story

My name is Austin and I am a second phase, Resident Assistant at TLC. I am twenty six years old and finally saved! It has been a long journey to reach the point that I'm at today.

I was raised in the Roman Catholic Church in Northern New Jersey, but my religion meant nothing to me except that I was pleasing my parents. At the age of thirteen I received my Confirmation, and that was the end of my road as a Catholic. At this age I was introduced to marijuana and alcohol, and I quickly developed a passion for the "party life." I was able to manage my academics along with my social life, so I was never too concerned about my substance abuse; I figured this was just a part of life as a teenager. Throughout high school I experimented with a variety of club drugs and hallucinogens, but I didn't get out of hand with these.

I went to Rutgers University from 2001-2006, and during these years of my life I spent days on end at clubs, raves, house parties, and any kind of social gathering I could find. In addition, I sold all sorts of drugs at school to support my lavish lifestyle. Nothing else mattered. Somehow I was able to graduate with a bachelor's degree in 2006. I thought my party life would fade away as I moved on in life, but it ended up taking a turn for the worse later on.

After I graduated college, I got a job with the Family Law Firm in Hackensack, NJ and worked for them as a paralegal for about two years. During this time, however, I had a severe opiate addiction that progressed from prescription drugs to heroin. Eventually, I had to resort to embezzling money from the office to support my addiction. I felt so alone and hopeless during these times of darkness. The lifestyle finally caught up with me, and I lost everything: my job, my apartment, my income, support from my family, and all hope in myself. Finally, in June of 2009 I decided to surrender and was brought to TLC by a family friend.

That same month I accepted Christ into my life, and I haven't been the same since. I now have an inner-peace, which I cherish whole-heartedly. I am filled with joy and gratitude for all Christ has done for me! I have hope for a prosperous future in which I will continue to serve Christ and carry out God's will for my life. Currently, I coordinate the Community Awareness ministry and facilitate a class for the residents on "Becoming a Contagious Christian." I am researching through many missionary organizations around the world, and I look forward to devoting the next couple years sharing God's love with others and expanding His kingdom with one of these organizations. Furthermore, my relationship with my family has been restored, and I have been blessed with unconditional love and support from my new friends and family in Christ!

Drinking in God's Word

Adam's Story

I grew up with a loving mother and father, but we didn't attend church, except on holidays. My mother was strict, and she cared about who I hung out with. My father was a sneaky alcoholic; he drank on the sly. He was also diagnosed bipolar and schizophrenic. Even though he was sick, he had a love for Christ. However, my parents divorced when I was eleven because of his drinking.

Once my father left, my rebellion kicked in. My dad had an apartment and I visited him. One day, he stopped at a bar to pick me up and had a bad accident. It terrified me. My mother notified me that it was due to drinking. Without my dad for a father figure, I ran amuck with my mother. I loved hanging out with the families that didn't care about their kids getting home on time. I started drinking and smoking pot at age thirteen with them, and everything else fell right into place. I had the mindset of a rebellious teenager.

At fifty-four, my dad packed up and went to Florida then got rebabtized and recommitted his life to Christ. For four months he had a good relationship with the church. He was four months clean. One day doing masonry work, he fell off a ladder and went into a coma for four days. We went to visit him, and all the people from church came to see him also. We were comforted with the people there. After the third day we left, and at this point my step-father and mother realized they had something missing, and they came to the Lord. My father passed away the day after.

I began to become very depressed. I got heavily into drinking and started to become the drinker who broke things and made a mess. I was still living with my mom, and she married my stepfather after my dad died. I continued to rebel. I tried to find women and use pot to fill the void. I didn't enjoy being with myself.

After high school, I went to culinary school and the Culinary Institute of America. I graduated in 2006 by the skin of my teeth. The week before I graduated, I flipped a jeep. The right side of my brain was bruised, and I was in ICU for six days and unconscious for six hours. My head was crushed, and I was saved because I had my seat belt on and was intoxicated, which made me relaxed. Still, they didn't know if I would be able to walk. During this time in school I had been doing a lot of drugs—mushrooms, cocaine, ecstasy. I lived next to Paterson NJ, but was fortunate that I never got into crack or heroin.

Slowly but surely, I was working my way back to drinking, starting with beer. I always had a reason why, a justification. I told myself I worked seventy-eight hours a week and needed to relax. I continued to work at Hackensack University Medical Center as a chef, then the Brownstone and the Pluckemin Inn, a four star restaurant. By then I had to start dealing with the repercussions of my accident. I was expelled from driving in NY for a year, and I hired an attorney. My NJ license was suspended a year and a half after the accident.

In order to get to work, my girlfriend decided that we would move within four miles of the restaurant. We got an apartment together, and we were engaged. My parents thought it was a good idea for me to be in a place of my own. My girlfriend worked 9-5, and I worked 11-11, so I started drinking behind her back. I drank all day at work. She would come home and smoke pot with me, and I'd continue drinking. In 2005 I was diagnosed bipolar, so I was on five medications and drinking at that same time, as if trying to commit suicide. I felt stuck in a ball and chain to alcohol. I didn't want to wake up.

I began stealing liquor, hiding bottles at home and work, I would get pain killers from work, and pot was like tobacco to me. I was numb—a slave to alcohol. I could not function without it. I was such a functional alcoholic; no one could compete with me at work. But then after a year and a half, they smelled liquor on me, and in less than a month from the wedding, I was fired. I had no job.

I had to explain to my fiancé why I lost my job. It was the first time I had ever been fired. We had to get rid of the apartment, and I had to move back in with mom and dad. The wedding was still on, so I found a four day job for a PGA golf tournament in Paramus, NJ.

My first day I set up in a clubhouse with the bar, and I worked without having a drink. On the second day, I worked twelve hours. Then the bar tender asked if I wanted a drink, and I had a twelve pack. By the third day, he was handing me coffee cups of vodka. I had sixteen coffee cups of vodka on the fourth day. People were buying me shots, but I didn't get caught. I was very sneaky—lying, cheating, and smoking cigarettes to cover up the smell of booze. I'm so personable and a schmoozer. People couldn't tell I was drunk. At the end of the day, I stumbled out to my car, got in, and passed out.

Management just happened to pass by my car and saw me passed out. A manager banged on the window, and I started fighting with the guy saying, "I'm all right," but I wasn't. He convinced me to turn the car off and offered to drive me home. He drove me home and everyone was there. All three saw me in my drunkest state. My fiancé said, "The wedding is postponed. You need help." I had to go to an outpatient program, AA, daily.

I stayed sober for five days and then was sneaking bottles of wine from my mom, the cheap stuff that was left over after my mom had thrown out the good wine. A couple of days after that, my mom had a brain aneurysm and died at age fifty-one. She had no previous medical problems. After that news, I switched from whiskey to Vodka. It had less of a scent. I isolated myself, lied, and showed up to the outpatient program—drunk. They sent me away to a twenty-eight day program in NJ.

I was too busy smoking cigarettes and staring at the girls to learn anything. I thought I'd just attend AA for the rest of my life. I came home and started looking for a job. Being home without my real parents, I started stealing pain killers from my step-father and quarters to buy liquor. By the fifth day, my step-dad was onto what I was doing. For two days he tried to get a bed for me at TLC. That night my fiancé and I had a terrible fight. The next morning, I woke up after the explosion, and my fiancé was gone.

I heard my step-father on the phone saying, "I need him out of the house." I left the house and wrote a note, "I love this family too much to cause any more pain." I knew I needed to go. I went three towns away to get the cheapest liquor. I kept getting messages on my cell phone, and I felt convicted. I took the first sip and felt really stupid. I called my step-dad and said I'd be home. I talked to my mom's friend from church. Forty-five minutes later my step father said, "Pack your bags, you're going to live with your sister."

The next day my fiancé called my sister. She contacted Owen Kelly from church to get me into TLC. I looked at the program on-line and said, "No way." I went to talk to Owen Kelly to tell him I didn't want to go. After talking to him, I was selling him the idea of how bad I needed to go. While I was with him, he called the director and told him about me, and the director replied, "I was praying for him." He said there's a bed open for me because my step-father's friend, Vinnie Barry, saw the director and asked for prayer and a placement for me.

I said to myself, "This is no coincidence." God needed me here. I started to believe God was who He said He was. I still thought it was a big joke at first. I took it for granted. I wanted to tell them how to help me. I ran my own program. I didn't trust and obey. He allowed me to fall again. I hit rock bottom and that rock was Christ. I relapsed in January of 2009 while working on the Community Awareness tables. It was my first day out there, and I shut my common sense off. I said to myself, "I'll have just one." I had a twelve pack, so they put me out of the program.

I had to wait a month to get back into TLC. They had me start all over with the program because I was still struggling with tobacco addiction. I fell in that area. Since I was already under grace, coming back into the program after what I had done, I had to go to the Mission in Albany, NY for thirty days. I needed to be there. My family didn't want me home, and I needed to see men dope sick— "Having the opportunity to drink and drug everyday scared the hell out of me."

Before I left there, I stumbled upon Jeremiah 29:11: "'For I know the plans I have for you,'" declares the Lord," 'plans to prosper you and not to harm you, plans to give you hope and a future.'" Even through my stupidity and rebellion, the Lord still had a plan for me. He grabbed a hold of me and carried me through. I came back thirty days later a different person. I was so happy to be back at TLC because there's something about this place, beyond the camaraderie, beyond the rules, beyond the love... There is a presence of Christ here.

When I came back to TLC, I had to start all over, and I was fine with that. I had a new attitude, a new a peace, a taste of Christ. I couldn't stop going after Him. The world views TLC as an escape from drugs and alcohol. But once you're clean, you find out it's a discipleship program. The Lord calls you out from the world to further his kingdom and to transform the world. I now know I cannot succeed without leaning on Christ for the rest of my days. All glory and honor to my Lord, Jesus Christ.